ALMOST NORMAL

By Ann Kolsrud

'One million people commit suicide every year'
The World Health Organization

Ann Kolsrud

Published by
Chipmunkapublishing
PO Box 6872
Brentwood
Essex CM13 1ZT
United Kingdom

http://www.chipmunkapublishing.com

Edited by Jurita Bennett and Mary Dow

Cover Image: By Laura Malm

ALMOST NORMAL

thankful to few

sorry to only one-- Jen

Ann Kolsrud

ALMOST NORMAL

Chapter One

My parents aborted me when I was twenty-six. I was a year short of being the same age as the other great artists like Morrison and Joplin who seemed to die prematurely. But unlike them, I was never known. I was a voice never heard, perceived or understood. But I could always hear myself. Why didn't anyone else, I wonder? Perhaps it was just that mine was a voice no one wanted to hear.

In the beginning, I was born in America in the state of awareness. The first thing which I became aware of was pain. The first doctor in my life slapped me on the butt and made me cry. His name was Dr. Tork. I always remembered his name because it rhymed with "stork," that great big bird whose purpose in life was to drop a "bundle of joy" upon a family's doorstep. But that bird also left a big mess to clean when people were not looking up, unprepared to catch the weight of a life, which had been delivered to them. Sometimes I have wished that the big white bird had a return address.

It was this weight that my parents caught, early on, and for which they signed. It was this fragile package that they held firmly within their protective arms. With great effort and want, I had been created. Everything that could insure pregnancy had been attempted- including a fertility specialist. It appeared that my parents were deserving of a child, for they had already owned a dog for years- which in America, seems to be a more accurate reflection of success than the number of children you own. In America the government will give you tax breaks for having children, and send them to school to get them out of your hair. If your children are hungry, the family can get financial help. In addition, most places of residence allow children. None of this applies to owning a dog. Even if you can afford one, and own one, sooner or later a neighbour will complain about the barking and take your dog away. Because of this, I still believe that the true measure of success is having a dog. But I have never quite figured out why it is easier to be a guardian of "man," than it is to be a guardian of "man's best friend."

My parents' dog was a silver-sable German-Shepherd named "Psych." Psych was my best friend. I use to stick my head in her food bowl when she was eating. At first, she wouldn't trust me and would growl, but I wasn't scared. I knew she wouldn't hurt me. Slowly she began to trust me and knew that I wasn't trying to take anything from her. I loved her so much that besides letting me comb and pet her, she would protect me.

ALMOST NORMAL

Then one day, I woke up and my parents told me that she was gone- they had aborted her first.

***

In this place, I am not afraid. I know I won't be hurt. Pain is relative to experience. Nothing can compare to the injury, which caused me to leave your world. My senses have been deadened, and the only thing that I am allowed to feel is this place.

***

So they made the transition from a four-legged animal to one that they hoped, one day, would walk on its own two feet. It appeared that their wishes had come true; they had a healthy baby. For some reason they didn't have any other babies besides me. Whatever the reason, it was good.

***

Here, it seems, on disability, all that is produced is bad. Of course, this is my critique of the film. People on the outside only look at the props, laugh, and then say I've got it good; the movie has become reality. The audience continues to think the actors are over-paid. I attempted to go on strike, but then I found out that I had unknowingly signed a contract -- with hell. It is not a comedy, but rather a film of horror.

**

My father had always been classified as an educator. So when people would ask what my father did for work; I would say he was in education. It seemed simple enough; that's what he said he was, so that's what he was. Whether they believed it, I do not know. He was a teacher to many, but a student to few; he had refused to take the tests with which I had challenged him.

My mother, on the other hand, was a princess, but no one else was really aware of this. My father had met this beautiful, blonde maiden on her island, which was surrounded by the leaking oil from her 58' Corvette. She got rid of the car after she married my father, but she never did leave her island.

**

What time is it? Time is not linear here. There is no value behind words such as hour, minute, even day. I can't go anywhere that I want to be, and there is no such thing as money. I'm just here, now that I no longer exist. I was sentenced to this place because I was unwanted.

ALMOST NORMAL

I guess, I could say it was June, and it would be June. I always liked June, because it was when I entered your world, and seemed to have a chance. But I never did; I had been conceived in the fall after the heat of the "Summer of Love" had dissipated.

Chapter Two

When I was five, I rode the big bus with smelly vinyl seats to a little building that was located out in the country. The smell reminded me of the time I got car sick. So every morning I did everything I could do to not heave and maintain myself.

The yellow, over-crowded, potential death-trap was my first connection to an educational system that was outside of my home. The government had herded us into this bus as if we were cattle - they called it a "busing shortage." The seats were only to be filled to capacity which left, at least, another four students standing. But who got to sit, and who remained standing was not based on fairness. It was purely chance. The large kids had an advantage because of their size. It seemed that they always had a place to sit. It was usually the younger kids, like me, who were not successful. A few times I was lucky, and the older kids would let me sit by them. So I would sit and watch the others who were left standing. The students sitting down usually found something about the seat-less to taunt and tease.

A person without a place was considered a loser. The other kids would say, "Hey loser, look at her clothes, is a flood coming?" A few times, I too, had to endure the focus of attention because there was no place for me and it made me cry. I didn't understand why they wouldn't let me just sit on the edge of one of the seats. I would have preferred the possibility of falling to the constant, prodding eyes of the winners.

Whether we were winners or losers, we always made it to our final destination. The older kids were usually dropped off first, at their building, and then we nervously awaited our arrival, fearful of the results to the tests we may have taken, and the new things we must learn in order to be accepted into the next grade.

The bus always pulled right up next to the building to drop us off, so we wouldn't have to cross the highway; the cars went by so fast. When the driver said it was okay for us to get up, we did. If the weather was nice, the teacher stood outside to greet us. I would watch her as I descended the steps of the bus into her control. It was here that they first tried to fix me.

***

I remember that in your world, everything used to break and needed fixing. It was ruled by entropy: the law of increasing disorder. But where I am now, wherever that is, nothing can be fixed. However you arrive in this position, nothingness is all you have until something changes - if it ever would. It really doesn't matter if things are broken. Things can't be fixed. At one time, I learned to accept this, and now I just don't feel anything. But don't get me wrong. Just because I have no feeling in regards to fixing things, doesn't mean I feel nothing at all. I do feel something. But I only have one feeling. I call it "this place." It's a feeling you don't have when you're alive and in your world.

***

They took me to a doctor. He ran a few tests. My parents replaced my presence to consult with him, and I was sent to the waiting room. I waited. I picked up a magazine about snakes, and just stared at the creatures that people so much feared. There were pictures of two snakes which looked similar. One was dangerous while the other was not. Most people couldn't tell the difference unless they looked very closely. I wondered if the doctor really could see me.

My parents eventually came out of the room. The doctor had given his opinion, and my parents had listened. The towering, stoic figures approached me with deliberation on their faces. They were determined to discover a way in which to plant the seeds of conformity in my mind.

This period of my education was defined as

ALMOST NORMAL

Kindergarten; it was the place they first tried to plant within me seeds for being a future member of society. The social aspect of school was rather a drag.

I wanted to learn. I excelled at everything I could. Recess, I always tried to dodge so I could stay inside and do independent learning activities. If they forced me outside, I hung around the trees and watched the ants skilfully ascend the bark. These trees were great big oaks. Their mighty branches seemed to dance, reaching up to the sky as if to catch something. The other children were not my friends. The only time they wanted to be around me is when they didn't understand something, usually to copy. All they wanted to do was play house, or some sports in which I found no interest.

It had always been acceptable to be myself until they had taken me to that doctor. After that, the teachers watched me. Everyone began to watch me from afar. Only the trees were my friends.

***

Now, I have no friends. All the people that I knew, like me, no longer exist. They flew crooked into a radiator of despair and suffering. I don't know if they chose that path, but I did. It was the best thing that could have happened. If we had tried to out-run the machine which was pursuing us, we would not have died with dignity. With broken legs from our futile attempts to escape, we would have crawled off the road, waiting to hitch-hike a ride from death that was still miles away...

***

In this place you don't age, at least mentally. I arrived when I was 26 so I am still the same age. My body is rotting though, actually quite fast. They didn't bury me very deep. Someday the top soil will wash away and others like me will emerge again. Either your kind will have to do something new or bury us deeper. Soon though, nothing will be left but bones.

Here, it's usually dark. It doesn't matter if you can see or not. Somehow you must fight yourself through a maze. As I struggle within, I find myself reaching out, feeling my way, trying to get to the end. But I'm starting to wonder if there is an end. Sometimes people give me advice and I dig and dig until my hands bleed. A few times, I have dug and seen daylight, but then the dirt starts to cave in on me, and I suffocate. I've even tried to scream, hoping someone would come rescue me. But unfortunately, no one seems to hear me, or they don't have the energy to dig me up, or they don't care.

ALMOST NORMAL

***

When I wasn't at school, I liked to hang out in the woods behind our house. It was mostly pine trees. The woods had originally been a lot for Christmas trees. Now these trees were much too big for any average house. And because no one had ever expected them to get that big, they were just smothering each other in their unnatural, human-sanctioned, growing space. I must have spent hours among them. When I was very little, I would walk up and down the aisles they formed. Here, I felt like the princess my mother was. I could imagine a great red carpet which honoured my feet with every step. As I got bigger, I tried to climb the trees. Soon I was a master. I scaled the trees with the ability of an ant, the ability I had so much admired. But I achieved true superiority when I dared to believe I was something that I was not.

I had not only marvelled at the ants, I had also been fascinated with the birds. Were they truly as free as they seemed? Many trees I had climbed had nests, and I was always careful not to touch the eggs. My mother warned me that if I did, the mother would not come back and be there for her young; I thought this was the most horrid thing which could happen to a little bird. If she did come back, she would treat them differently. I didn't think this would be much better. So with great reverence to the nests, I climbed and began to imagine I was a bird.

As I stood on the highest branch of the tallest tree, I stretched my small arms out into the big sky. With complete belief in what I was doing, I took a mighty leap straight into the arms of the tree in front of me. I began to imagine I was a bird. Soon, it seemed that no matter how far the tree was in front of me, I could make it. I could fly!

Everyday I could, I went to the woods to be anointed. Upon my return, there would always be sap in my hair, sap on my clothes, along with the occasional tick which had to be removed. My mother, despite all the mess it created for her, allowed me to go to the woods. I belonged there, and I was safe; I never got hurt. I had so much fun with the trees. I only wish that they could have talked.

***

Here I am free. It doesn't matter what I say or do. It doesn't matter; there is no punishment worse than being here. Only God is my authority; but even a higher power, I've come to question. Would my creator have allowed me to suffer so much? But it doesn't matter, I no longer suffer. I feel so many emotions at the same time; everything seems to balance, resulting in the

ALMOST NORMAL

formation of a being completely numb and non-living. I am happy that I am free but freedom has its price. I have become a non-person.

Chapter Three

Elementary school was just an extension of Kindergarten. At first, they didn't try to change me. I continued to dodge recess if I could, but I wasn't very successful. So I hung out with the only friend I had. It was all right, it passed the time, but I hated it. Soon she became bored with the monotony of my activities, and decided to spread out into new territory, which meant other people. Unfortunately there were no trees in which to shelter myself from my projecting loneliness. So not to call attention to myself, lest they try to fix me one more time, I forced myself to be something I wasn't, and knew that I wasn't.

Thinking of the situation, the term "hunting" comes to mind. I was starving for friends, or for at least to appear that I had friends. In what position of the social ladder, did I belong? I had to hunt down the people that would be with me. So with bow and arrow in hand, I shot down two easy targets - a couple of loners. At first they were just my catch, or rather, prize which I sported along my sides. I never wanted to hurt them, and never did. They were just the game that I had won, the trophies at my side which suggested I was a winner. But the truth is that the hunted had saved the hunter, and these people soon became my friends.

ALMOST NORMAL

Every year, I prepared for the hunt. And through this process my friends would appear through the camouflage. I became increasingly skilled as a hunter and captured more and more friends. But I began to desire to be hunted myself; they should come to me.

In the fourth grade, I was transferred to another school. I made a few friends, but a lot of enemies. Now not only did the teachers know that I was "different," but also the students with their increasingly, clearer perception of weirdness. I tried to look like I "fit in," but no one could close their eyes to my dishevelled appearance. I took great pain in choosing between the two sweatshirts I had to wear in which to keep myself warm. Would they notice that I had been wearing the same sweatshirt three days in a row? I carefully planned how to alternate between the two, hoping that it was enough change to leave everyone unaware. But as I tried to keep myself warm a chill surrounded me; everyone had noticed and they began to point fingers - at me! I was responsible for my poor hygiene: I wore the same clothes every day. But no one cared to know that these were my only warm clothes. It was my fault for wearing the same thing each day; my parents would provide for me. This was so far from the truth. But because the truth stood at such a great distance people could see what they wanted to believe. I then continued to breathe within a hallucination of mis-belief, being further misunderstood.

***

My father says I'm hallucinating, or rather that I am just twisted. Where I got such ideas he doesn't know. But what he doesn't know is that I try to tell myself that these things are made up, and that they couldn't be real.

So when my Grandmother tells me the story about a little girl in paper-thin clothing freezing at the bus-stop, I remind myself that this is just a story. But when potential frost bite begins to lick me, I can taste a memory too powerful to deny. So as she continues with the story, I continue to remember. It was my grandparents who bought me a coat. But within this package of warmth, was even more coldness. To ensure that I would not quickly out-grow the waist-length coat, it was purchased to hang below my knees. So every day I had to make a choice; would I rather freeze or be tortured with ridicule? I learned at an early age that decisions were not always easy.

I wore the coat from fourth grade until tenth grade. This was not my decision. My mother looks back at this clothing marathon, running at the mouth to everyone about their *poor* child. I don't understand but she wears my experience like some badge of honour.

ALMOST NORMAL

***

The distance at which they began to place me increased. It was too far to walk. Each year the distance increased. I now needed a car to catch up. I didn't know how to drive, but despite the fact that I was too young, I was going to learn.

I got into my car, and tried to position myself, but it was no use, I didn't fit. Slowly under the discerning eye of the teacher, I put my feet up on the sides of the desk, and leaned back in my chair, cruising down my own private road. Suddenly, there she was on private property. "Should I run her down?" I thought to myself. I wasn't going to slow down; I was already too far behind. Suddenly she was there. Her mighty force tried to mould me into shape, and then I crashed.

Soon I found myself surrounded by a curious crowd. They said my hand had crashed right into the face of the teacher. No one seemed to care that she had kicked me, denting me even more. But to this, there were no witnesses, and because of this, no one was going to listen to me. So for an hour a week I was sent to another institution.

The people there wanted to talk to me - there had

to be some catch. Sure enough, they were being paid to listen. I thought it should be the other way around; I should be paid to talk. I believe my parents began to think that wouldn't have been such a bad idea, after the number of uneventful sessions, which produced only a few "yes's" and "no's."

My parents throughout the accident were concerned, but for whom, I'm not sure. My father was a well-known, local educator. Possibly this could have been a reflection of his true ability to work, and not the show everyone thought they were seeing. So in order to tame the tiger that had started to bite, he got out his whip, and started whipping the beast which he had brought into this world. Scars formed without any wounds. With incredible stoicism, my father had attempted to carve conformity into my mind with his words. I was given a piece of paper stating various do's and don'ts. To honour my father, I only had to obey them. In addition to this, the paper contained an outline of my expected activities for every minute. The whole thing was rather ridiculous, and destined to fail. Not only had I thought this, but my parents also. Soon it was forgotten. I returned to school. The damage seemed to be repaired, and insurance had covered it. The New Year began, and life was moving smoothly.

ALMOST NORMAL

Now I was approaching Junior High. I needed my mother. I decided to trade my car in for a canoe, and paddled, fighting the current to reach her. But it was no use. She was too busy with "things." With great tenacity I finally made it to shore, only to find out that she couldn't help me anyway. The many years of seclusion on her island left her incapable of helping me. But I thought I could try to let her help me.

She took me into a room, and showed me her closet. There were out-dated shoes in rows along the closet floor beneath the clothing which seemed to be continuously pressed, because of the huge volume and little space. As I waited for an explosion, she reached in and relieved some of the pressure. Pulling out a dress that had pictures of turtles on it, she said, "I've had this dress since eighth grade."

I began to feel nauseated. Was this the only person I had to help me learn to dress like a female? I walked to my room, and started to feel a little better. I then realised it had been the overwhelming smell of moth-balls that had made me sick. I began to wonder if there was any way to enliven the clothing that had been laid to rest, and so carefully embalmed, so many years ago.

But the fact remained; I didn't have many clothes, or even the know-how to put these limited pieces together. My mother, admitting I had a clothing shortage, volunteered to take me shopping. Shopping for my so-called "new" clothes led me down the back alleys to where I witnessed poverty for the first time.

The Mission and St. Vincent de Paul's became the establishments frequented in attempting to clothe me. Some of the stuff wasn't all bad but most of it wasn't what I would choose to wear. I didn't understand why we had to shop there. It wasn't that my parents were hard up for money.

But my mother was a princess, and this was her flower garden. She liked to go and fight through the weeds to find that blooming item. She found a few furs, in which to encase her royalty. The animal which had worn these furs had been gone a long time, but not as long as my mother.

***

I wish I had a fur. Sometimes it gets so cold. They must be waiting to identify me. Maybe someday they'll open the door and pull my tray out. Will anyone that I knew before recognize me? The clothes I wear here are wearing away; soon they'll be in shreds like the life I had worn. But sometimes, it also gets so hot that I can imagine myself outside the oven of a crematory. I wish I could open a window. But either there isn't one, or they are frozen shut by the cold, unconcerned stares of the people on the outside who do not understand. I won't complain; it wouldn't do any good. I tried one time, but the attendant said the conditions were acceptable. Sometimes I forget, and must keep reminding myself that I am no longer alive.

***

Junior High was just a school for children whom had grown a little too big for their desks. This is where I truly started to realize that I looked as out of place as my mother would if she were to leave her island. It was very hard to try and fit in. All the other girls always looked so pretty. I felt like the ugly duckling, but the truth was I simply looked like a boy. My parents had this idea that I had rejected the idea of being a girl. This was not true. It was just that the only female in my life was gone most of the time, searching for new things to place in the gardens around her castle.

My father worked very hard while my mother sat on her throne. Both of them were very busy. But it seemed if anyone was capable of spending some time with me, it would be my father. Every night his tired body entered the front door, but only on occasion did he come home.

When my mother was home, she attempted

to clean. Seconds, minutes, hours, and eventually the day passed, but her cleaning never ended - or rather, never really started. Her few seconds of distraction from her work progressed the same way: seconds to minutes, minutes to hours. Some days, nothing had been accomplished. But it was during these "breaks" in which my mother arose, so high above her throne, neglecting her kingdom, that she released me to the world she had so long ago escaped.

Suddenly I found myself embraced by the loving sounds of music. And through these sounds were messages of other kingdoms, in which I knew my mother longed to be. I would look up at my mother's face, and I knew that she had arrived; her imagination had become reality. She now was too far away to be reached; I could not reach that high. But now she could never leave me; we had found common ground. We would forever be connected, on our appreciation of worlds beyond our own.

After her attempted escapes, my mother was always very tired. She would then lie down, to read the daily newspapers. But similar to her cleaning, she never finished reading them; so they would lie in piles forming towering cities of their own. She attempted to finish them but after reading a few lines, she was once again, far away, in another world of dreams.

ALMOST NORMAL

***

I cannot dream, nor can I imagine, or escape. I seem to be frozen here. They shot a lot of chemicals into my blood stream, attempting to reanimate me, but it failed; it only seems to have created further damage. Someday they will have the technology to bring me back to life. But for now, the government spends thousands of dollars in maintenance costs, trying to bring me forward by bringing me back into the world which rejected me.

***

My mother sometimes stood up and attempted to walk down uncarpeted aisles, but she would always return to her natural position. When I was a baby she would hold me up close in her arms as she sat in her chair. But as I got bigger, she could no longer hold me, and I had to stand at her side. Even though I had grown quite tall, it didn't matter; because of the incredible height at which she sat, she could only notice me when she was looking down.

The few years had made me a lot bigger. I was now in Junior High and big enough to crawl out of my window at night. At one a.m., out the window I went, a thief in the night attempting to break into a reality outside my home. I walked about a mile to meet my friends. We had fun just pondering the concept of rebellion. But soon after, the concept was conceived, and delinquents were born. After a few broken windows and spray-painted houses, we were named. Then without warning, our movements were terminated - quickly and quietly. I didn't realise my parents knew anything about my sleeping habits until I had tried to leave, and my windows would not open - they were nailed shut.

Then there was the mini-bike. Everyone else in the area had one, and my parents, trying to make me happy, purchased one for me. I loved riding. It seemed that for the first time I was in control of my destination. I thought I was free. I soon found out I wasn't.

The bike I had was an off-road bike. My friends and I challenged this limitation, and flew up and down the paved streets. We were still careful though, and never strayed too far onto the main roads, the roads on which we did not belong. But one day the line of division faded for me, and I suddenly found myself way over the edge.

It had just been one of those days: so free of the confining cage, without clipped wings. With my friend on back, I had taken flight down the roads of uncertainty. Suddenly a car had appeared, and the red vultures which circled above it began to chase us down. I flew, speeding down the roads, unaware of the signs with no destination in sight. Finally, the lines of limitations captured me in their net. Exhausted from my futile attempt at escape, I surrendered to the impending feast. I must have already been dead, so why had I attempted to flee?

I had dared to fly further than I could, and suddenly I had landed short of my destination, and in court. At twelve years of age, I had broken more traffic violations than an average person would in a life time. So it was back to school for me. I obviously had missed something somewhere. And in fact, that's what they did. They sent me back to Kindergarten. The place that had sent me away to be fixed was now fixing people. The old school house in the country was now the court house. Once again, I would be judged.

***

Even though I've been sentenced to this place, I will never leave the court room. The judge has left, but the court room still has its own opinion. It doesn't matter that I'm dead and, also, certified not guilty. They continue to search for an explanation to something they do not understand.

Ann Kolsrud

The question which torments them only continues to prevent me from resting in peace: how could this have happened to someone so young, so pretty, and so intelligent? To resolve this dilemma, they have found blame. It is my fault! I am guilty.

***

I had gotten off easy that time. I only lost a small part of my freedom; I had to sell the bike. Back in my parent's cage I went, and there I remained with newly-clipped wings.

The next year passed without incident: good grades, good behaviour. It appeared to be the beginning to a shiny, promising future; but the shadows were slowly descending on my horizon, to create a future which promised to insidiously come to an end.

***

I like to visit my grave sometimes. It's still there, though it's only marked by some ambiguous, nine-digit, number; my name has been forgotten. I guess that's the interesting part of it. They could know almost everything about me if they wanted, but they choose not. Maybe if they were interested, they would know that I don't belong here; I am innocent. But instead, they just

ALMOST NORMAL

keep planting flowers on the surface, in the dirt
which covers my rotting corpse.

Chapter Four

The beginning of high school was going to be a beginning to a new life. It was all there in my head. I imagined it, I could conceive it, but would it be achieved? After all, my father was now, not just an educator, he was the principal of my high school. All the kids (at least a majority) thought he was "cool." I thought it would be so perfect if I could be just as cool and as accepted as my father. So I spent countless hours ruminating about an unreality that seemed possible.

The school year began, and yes, everyone did come to me - they were afraid. They wanted to share the knowledge I possessed about the workings of yet another part of an institution which I had grown up around. One by one they came for my advice, and one by one they left never to return; I was only valuable when I was needed.

But that's what I had expected, and now I would go on with my life. I was a super-achiever; I was in music, sports, and all the honours classes while maintaining my 4.0. Only three freshmen had been chosen for the jazz band, and of course I was one. And though I was never a runner with innate talent, circumstances would allow it that I got to run varsity my first year. I liked cross-country and track because I could run for my own pursuits; I was never a team player. So this was my life, at least I controlled it, and it would not leave me- so I thought. But I did not expect that my life would find that I was not needed, and also leave me.

***

I hope that someone would see I was out of place, and not leave me to fend for myself. Would they know that I was not well even if I could smile and tell them that I needed help? I fear that they would not help me unless my pleading for help was within conversations with myself and if I ran from them as they tried to listen in.

***

But before this would happen, I would walk on a cloud of optimism. Everything I "put my mind to," worked out, far beyond my expectations. And during this time, rays of love shined upon me; I could do no wrong.

Not only could I do no wrong, neither could anyone else. I attempted to do everything to the best of my ability, why couldn't anyone else? I was aware of the obvious "losers," the people who did not try. There seemed to me to be no excuse for their lack of dedication to learning. If I saw someone crying, I thought, "my God, what's their problem?" I didn't care to try to understand what was going on. I didn't ask; I didn't know. I would just look at them, and if they seemed to be some of those underachievers, I figured it was probably something mundane that they should get a grip on. It wasn't that I lacked the ability to care. It was just that I could handle my life, and I didn't understand why they couldn't. It was easy to see the frame, but I didn't get the picture. I didn't know the artist or the motivation behind this creation. I couldn't appreciate the work. This was not because I was uneducated; it was because I was just stupid. At least I could use my limited years as an excuse. I always wonder if God is punishing me for having been so cold and narrow-minded.

***

Here I hang on the wall of my limitations, fading from the light that shines upon my illusion of wellness. Sometimes, they turn off the light, and I am left alone. But when they come to view me, the light is always turned back on. A few are knowledgeable and can understand; They can appreciate my passion and struggle. But most, the "aesthetes," are truly ignorant, and find their interpretations by looking at the frame, the light, and then think that somehow, they could do better.

Last night, one particular gentleman whom I believed to be educated, came to my museum. He stared for a long time while announcing loudly

to the room that I was just a
waste of the tax payer's money.   He paid his
taxes, and wondered why he had to support this. I
agreed that some change was needed, for I was
fading in my current position. But, he just wanted
to cut the whole thing out. He would never allow
his work to hang here so why did I? I tried to tell
him that when you are a starving artist, and art
seems to be the only way in which you can feed
yourself, you can't choose. Choice is an illusion.
But he still could not understand or appreciate; he
too, was not part of the culturally elite. He was
just a person, a person who thought he "knew."

***

During this time my mother somewhat
shifted to the background, and I truly became my
father's daughter. I got along great with my family
when I got along great with my father. The
relationship with my family also improved when I
didn't need my mother; it wasn't good to place
"unnecessary" stress on her. It all seemed to be
working out.   Three more years, and I would
graduate, and go on to college to pursue medicine
or some other professional career.

***

They thought I would be good at mopping
floors, but I thought I would just get lost in the

circles which formed within the conversations with me. Round and round I would go, trying to find depth so I could somewhat escape the menial existence they had in mind for me. But there would be no actual physical escape. I would be trapped in a circumlocutory routine, locomoting every bone and fibre in my body to pull a weight of incredible loss; I think I can, I think I can - but I don't want to.

***

Suddenly, without warning, my cloud of optimism began to darken. I didn't know why. Suddenly things didn't work out with ease, and I felt sick all the time. It was in the middle of my sophomore year that it started to rain.

At school I was becoming very nervous; it was life or death whether I made it to my next class on time. The bell would ring and I would race to the finish line - the next class. I could feel my heart well up inside me as I ascended the mighty hills, to the top floor in which my next class was located. I was in an altered state; I was in tune to myself, while being fearfully aware of everything around me, lest something jump out and obstruct my path. I feared that I was different, and feared even more that everyone would pick up on this, and they did. They began to watch me, and I could see the malevolence which they harvested in their thoughts. Even though I was losing my mind, I continued to achieve but at a much slower pace than previously. I made it into National Honour Society, got on the student council, and at the same time, flunked a few classes. And with the close of each semester, and each year, there would be that same speech from my father, "This is not going to continue." His statement was accurate; it was going to get worse.

Before my senior year began, I got my first job. I was a receptionist for a veterinarian clinic. In addition to the receptionist's part, I cleaned, counted out medicines, and weighed animals. I liked the job, and it seemed to be working out. But one day, my boss pulled me into his office and said, "Some days you are just great, and other days, you walk around like a zombie - shape up or ship out."

I didn't realise I was this way. It had happened; something that I had put my mind to do, I couldn't do. I had always known there were some things I could not do, but this part-time job seemed tangible. My life was no longer in my control. I had failed, and I could not face my parents. So I ran away from home, and I haven't been back since.

***

Ann Kolsrud

I'm no longer running. I just sit on my butt, and fill out a lot of forms. It is a full time job. The job follows me everywhere; I not only take it home, it is my home. The pay sucks, and I'm embarrassed to tell people I do this for a living. Unfortunately I'm so dependent on the few benefits this position offers that I can't see looking for some other job. They encourage people to take an early retirement in what they call, "work incentive," but at the same time they do all they can to ensure that you will die doing the work that you were forced to do. I've tried everything to break the contract; but the only way to break this legal document is to do something illegal. I have considered this, but at this time I choose not to lower myself any more than I already am.

***

Soon after I had begun my senior year, I dropped out. I did not choose this, I just could not continue. For unknown reasons, the runner had collapsed, and was taken to the hospital - the mental hospital.

I appeared to most to be another troubled teenager. So carefully they analysed me, reducing me to a sophist; I existed, especially my problems, because of the environment, and people which surrounded me. First of course, it was me being a teenager, then my relationship with my father, then my relationship with my mother. Just before I thought they were going to ask if I had a dog, and whether or not I got along with it, they labelled me mentally ill.

They released me, and I went back to school. I took two classes in my senior year, in order to graduate. I finished and graduated - with honours. This was my last achievement in their world. My diploma was a simple piece of paper that authenticated an accomplishment.

***

He had given me a lot of paper. It too, acknowledged my success. I ran through the green fields of my new found success to the fine department stores. When I got tired I sat down to elegant dining, or perhaps, spent a night at the Broadmoor. Eventually I quit running through the fields, and drove my brand-new Honda Accord EX down the smooth pavement of respect. The grass grew so easily that I could not see the weeds. Other people seemed to be working hard. They would be out mowing, and the wind would just blow it into the streets. I drove through it, without a care in the world. I was successful and everyone knew it. They didn't care what I had actually accomplished.

Ann Kolsrud

Chapter Five

At the last minute, I applied for college. It was either go to school or get a job, neither of which I felt capable of doing. So I went to the college that my father had attended. Though I remained uncertain to what had actually happened to me in high school, I was determined to put the past behind me and be successful. I purchased my books and began reading them even before classes had begun. I was going to make it.

I started classes and attended them religiously. I did the usual school thing; I lived in a crappy, over-crowded dorm, consumed the infamous cafeteria food, and studied - occasionally. No matter how little I studied, I maintained good grades. The girl across the hall from me recognised this, and as if I possessed some great secret to academic performance, sought out my friendship. Soon Sherri and I were just great friends. We had a couple of the same classes. When we weren't in class we were together trying to find beer and pizza. She was the best friend I had ever had.

But soon the religion became routine, and down on my knees I went, without knowing why. Suddenly, I could no longer get up. I had to drop out of school. My mind remained frozen in prayer to the degree I wanted so much to obtain, but my body was shipped back to my parent's home.

I was put on more lobotomizing drugs, and then attended the college that was in my home town. It proceeded much the same way; I started out, stretching out into the myriad of opportunities which were available to me, only to curl up into the womb of torture which encased me.

Through some umbilical cord of sanity, I was able to complete a couple of classes. But soon the connection with this school would be severed. My father was being fucked professionally, and this pseudo sexual experience would deliver me miles away, to another state, and another school.

***

I had been delivered from empty hands; hands which could never hold my slippery weight. He alone, held me within his large welcoming hands. He accepted the responsibility, and carefully moulded me into a more functional presence. I was born into an unfamiliar world.

Suddenly there was a great light, I was cleaned, and then wrapped in a blanket of security. He took me home, and showed me off to a privileged few; the friends he could trust. I was his ward. It had all been fun, and exciting at first.

But the meconium appeared, forming something which he feared and could not tolerate. He then put me in a dumpster and closed the lid, never to be seen again.

***

My father got a new job, doing the same thing and my mother found a new place to sit. I too, found something new in which to do the same thing; I entered the local university, and dropped out.

I had been going to school when I suddenly ended up in another hospital. This hospital revered for its excellence, treated me by dumping medication into me. I became a human container of toxic waste. After being released, I staggered my way into a friend's car and was driven home.

I attempted to return to school but my eyes could not focus, and the lines and words which floated around the paper simply became too difficult to capture and understand. The sweat of exhaustion quickly evaporated, as did my desire to finish the race which had no foreseen finish line. So I stopped to rest drifting in and out of a form of coma. My mother would approach me, and feel my pulse to make sure I was still alive. Sometimes, I would rise, and attempt to walk through the doors which had suddenly appeared in the walls. Then as quick as they had appeared, they disappeared. The doors were gone, and I was completely surrounded by walls, alone, with only no way out. Once again I had ended up in the hospital- this time to be taken off the medication.

***

They say the reason the medicine never helped me very much is because I didn't give it a chance. They call this "noncompliance." But at first, the doctors were Gods; they were going to deliver me once again, but this time from my pain. They seemed safe and legitimate. I thought I wanted what they had to offer. The pills would make me "normal." They would open my eyes to all that I had been missing in my life. So believing this to be a good thing, I swallowed every pill, waiting for the fruitful results to follow. But all that this "original compliance" gave birth to was pain.

Ann Kolsrud

Chapter Six

I had entered a different hospital, for a slightly, different reason. This doctor, at least, seemed to care and listened intently trying to interpret the slurring words which emerged from my numb face. I would surface occasionally, to understand the words that were being said. As I left my first encounter with the psychiatrist, I bobbed back and forth through the hallway to the wing of recovery; hoping that I would be released from the hook of the drug-induced insanity which had captured me.

Eventually the drugs were reduced to a tolerable level, and I was released from the hospital. I was sent home to another confinement: the acidic restraints of a generation gap - my parents.

I was, now, too old to be at home. I was 19 and pursuing nothing but my sanity. I had begun to form my own opinions, interests, and wanted to disagree with my parents. The whole arrangement was a bad thing. The animals were placed in a way not sanctioned by nature with no one to entertain.

A typical day would be a boring day at the family's zoo. My father would entertain himself with the electronic buzz of visual dots as my mother would rise from her chair, and fly into a nest between the trees. I would sneak around the house without being detected. Casually I would slide from one dimension to another, fading in and out from one substance to another, only to end up with no other person than myself. But it all had its function. The more I wasn't noticed the more separate I could be from them, and the restraints which hungered to burn me if I attempted to escape conformity. Being so distant, I challenged myself to exist high on a hill, far from the corroding waters of the recent flood of hospitalisations. I felt so safe staring down into the streams, away from their touch. But despite my great effort, I was bound and gagged and plunged deep into the waters as a wave of sound pulled me along by the ear.

I had slowly gathered my senses together only to be overcome by the four octave screeching of Yma Sumac. I twisted in agony as ripples of loudness explored every corner of the silence I had found at the edge of my confinement.

Somehow I would find the key to unlock the restraints, and the cage in which I existed; I would connect to the outside. I knew though that my mother would destroy me for making another long distance call to a world which seemed so far away. But there would be no calls; the line would be silenced. It would no longer be needed because I would plant myself under the cool shade of a silver maple. I would live safely between the two worlds; blooming in the shadows, and fading in the sun. But as I began to take root once again, I was transplanted to the campus of yet another school.

***

I live in a zoo. But this is a different kind of zoo. No one would ever pay to visit it. But if they ever were to find themselves encaged and staring the animals in the face, then they would be sure to pay something - possibly their soul.

Once a month a few scraps are thrown into the cage, and the starving animals devour them within the first week. After that it's best to stay clear, or they will eat you alive. But after that, when there is nothing left to suppress the hunger which grows, they search for anything that will appease the satiety centre of their minds. If you happened to save a little, and they come knocking at your door, you must always say "no." Because once you feed a wild animal, it will come back and eventually become dependent on you. So I say "no" to their suffering eyes and watch them flee back into the human jungle.

***

So I attended another school. By now my

parents had started to "cut me off"; they attempted to sever the connection. Now I was attending a private, religious school. I entered the school wearing my black, leather jacket with a faded denim vest donned with Harley patches. The resident assistants had been forewarned of my mental difficulties, and I was escorted to my private cell.

This time I only pursued a status of part-time. I took three classes and got all A's. Apparently I learned something although it seemed so trivial compared to what I had begun to learn about human nature.

Once again I ended up in the hospital. This time they were determined to correct me. But before they could correct me, they had to know what was wrong; and so the lessons, the brain-washing, began.

***

A minister came to visit me in the hospital. He said that all I needed was to wash away the demons from my mind with prayer. So I held on tightly to his hands praying that this was all that I needed. We read the Bible; I surrendered my soul to God and waited for a miracle. Then the staff sent him away, and I returned to my room - still sick.

Ann Kolsrud

***

Now my doctor, the same doctor who had seemed to care, set me up with a social worker. This social worker specialized in treating people who had been sexually abused. The doctor was certain that she was going to figure out my problem. With her narrow tunnel of specialisation, she attempted to find and clear the blockage I possessed which had stymied my ability to function. Perhaps some hang-up within my personality was preventing me from flowing through life. But because of her "help," the only thing I came close to doing smoothly was being flushed down a toilet with my head full of shit.

Because I seemed so normal but was so dysfunctional, I was difficult to diagnose. I did not appear to be psychotic, so the mental health professionals began to believe that some horrible thing had happened to me; I was a product of abuse. So carefully, this social worker and I explored every experience that had occurred in my life. But still, I could recount nothing horrible. But because many abused people block out their memories of abuse, this social worker, this " therapist" forced her ideas down my throat, and I started to remember " things" that I could not remember; " things," which had never happened.

ALMOST NORMAL

First it was my high school boy friend who had abused me. Unfortunately, this point of view was too simple and did not explain problems which had occurred before this relationship. The cause of my problems remained blurry. So instead, this social worker began to focus on my father.

It seemed as if this was the perfect solution; my father was responsible for my insanity. If he had not hurt me I would be "normal." So relentlessly, I proceeded to question my mother. Eventually, I found that this line of questioning was ridiculous. My father had not "touched" me. The only thing which had touched me, that I had unknowingly allowed to touch me, was suggestion; I swirled, caught with the bowl of their diagnosis. It was easy for them to dump me in this category. But I would not flush; I clung to the rim of truth despite their attempts at "sanitisation." Soon they forgot the whole thing. I regained some strength, crawled out from the unseen forces of suggestion, and attached myself to the bottom of society - still sick.

***

People that reside above the bottom occasionally look down at the parasites which feed on them. With their judging, analytical eyes, the purveyors of the indigent expect to feed themselves on this obsequious fodder: gratitude, thankfulness, indebtedness, and so on... But so often their dinner is spoiled by an acerbic after-taste; the parasites refuse to "kiss-ass." They try to spit the taste out of their mouths, and cleanse themselves of the contact by distancing themselves from the encounter. So from a distance the people still await to taste the humbleness, or rather, humility, of the people on the bottom. The truth is that it is a symbiotic relationship; the people feed on each other.

I try to behave in a manner which I consider respectable. I do not desire any past episode of any intentional, inappropriateness to come knocking at my door, when, if ever, I have the opportunity to throw a party. But I am imperfect although it seems I am not human.

Everyday I look up to the functional world for support and guidance. The functional people who don't know of my situation treat me as an equal - with respect. I watch them with deep admiration, searching for some hint as to what makes them "able", and me "disabled." But the others who know of my bleak reality only enforce it; it's hard to look up when others are looking down and blocking my view.

People only can rise to a level near what is expected of them. Some may fall short of this expectation while others can far exceed it. Unfortunately for me, it seems the expectations allotted to the category in which I have been placed, only encourages me to stay at the bottom.

I possess the vocabulary of an abecedarian; however, if any terminology, especially that which, to some, borders on being grandiloquent, escapes my orifice, I am reprimanded. Either they castigate me for not fitting in the category to which I've been placed, or they do not understand and ask me to speak with a forced tongue; I must use the vocabulary of a child: see Jane run - from this?

If I am able to out-run this challenge, I still have to avoid the mines which are hidden in the field of benefits; for every step forward I must take at least two sideways. Despite this adversity, I continue to envision the hill on which I will place my flag.

Chapter Seven

When I first got on disability, I thought it was a great thing - I was a stupid kid. I got more money from the government than my parents. In fact, I had an opportunity to be independent from them. It was a simple existence; I went to college and lived like the majority of other poor students. I was reasonably content with my position. I wanted "more," but I didn't know exactly what that was.

My parents informed me that the semester which I was attending, would be the last that they would support, if I had to drop out. Half-way into the semester, I had to drop out; I had flunked the relatively, easy course of sanity, and instead, I was forced to pursue a career in psychology as a Guinea pig. Again, I had ended up in the hospital unaware of the tests to which I would be, subjected.

ALMOST NORMAL

Chapter Eight

I was once again in the hospital. It seemed to be part of the routine - in and out. It was a form of copulation which I thought at first to be safe. But the relationship was becoming stale, and I wanted somehow to end it. But like an addict, I could not stray too far from my addiction. There had to be a way out, but how? Soon the solution revealed itself to me; the protective barrier between the help and hurt began to strip away. One by one articles of clothing began to fall on the floor. It would be the start of an unprofessional relationship.

**

I once felt human with a lady I was seeing. But when her concern for me grew great they told her that she was "too emotionally involved." The next time I saw her she was so far away that I missed her. Then I began to forget that feelings were a part of being human.

**

I had been in the hospital, facing a transfer to the state hospital. This was not the solution I had been seeking. It was obvious that no one could help me, so I decided to leave. My trembling spirit gathered my things and left the institution which had failed me. There was no destination, except for the pay phone which stood out from the dark, overwhelming shadows of my surroundings.

I carefully looked up the doctor's name and number as the phone book trembled in my hands. I found the number, put the money in, dialled, and prayed that he would soon be on the other end. His number began to ring, my heart began to pound, and I could feel perspiration clinging to my forehead as I waited for the two ends to make a connection.

"Hello," he said. It was him. It was the voice I was so desperate to hear. He was my only hope.

"It's me," I said. That was all I could say. Those few words were suddenly somehow the extent of my entire vocabulary. All I could do was create some noise to suggest a "yes" or "no." I had come this far only to find myself suddenly paralysed, without words. I was completely vulnerable. He had the power to sever the connection, the umbilical cord to my life.

My fate was being delivered. I followed my fate, and drove down the new unfamiliar road to his home. It was then that he took me in, sheltering me from my fears and began to adopt me. I felt safe and secure in his home, and with him. I sat facing him, knowing that my life without him had ended, and wondering if I would have an opportunity to live.

He brought me back to life slowly introducing me to the world. At first the world seemed so ominous, and the burden of my weight too much for him to bear. I cried. I endeavoured indefatigably to learn to be the person he wanted me to be.

I was now out of school, searching aimlessly for a place to rest. During this time, I grew closer to him and further from my parents. My dependence for him started with an occasional twenty dollar bill, was followed by the dissolution of my disability benefits, and ended with my being completely dependent on him for all my needs. Soon the green spread as if it were some out of control weed: feeding on my insecurity and absorbing my autonomy. My new identity developed; I was primed and ready for show.

I had bloomed, and the love I felt for him did too. He was my mentor, my lover, and my friend. I was in love. He had rescued me. The great void in my life had been filled, and I towered above it, branching out to the life and opportunities around me. He was a God, he had made me.

Ann Kolsrud

As I grew closer to him, my love for him took root and grew deeper. I even loved his imperfections - they were perfect. But the more I loved him; the less I loved myself. Suddenly I found myself entangled in confusion, struggling to understand my identity. Who did he love, I wondered? Was it my beauty or my person? So as I laboured to be beautiful, carefully painting my face to display the illusion, he would look the other way. The illusion suggested innocence so easily removed. And fearing his effect on such a creature, he ordered me to remove the paint. I then looked into his eyes, and I could see an aging man frightened within. It was youth he feared.

***

The greatest difficulty is that I am torn between two worlds. I have my friends that do lunch with the elite or functional people of society, and then I have my friends from the human jungle. It seems unnatural that a person could witness such extremes; one person to feel the flesh gripped and pulled in two different directions. The question presented is "Which world do I live in? " There are the memories of being on top, but the truth is I have been pulled underwater to drown. My occasional contact with people on top is just my bobbing for air. I hate to think what would happen if they suddenly grew tired of me and quit coming around.

***

I was someone, someone special. I was living with a dream that had put to sleep the old tiring struggle, and awakened the sleeping doors which before had been closed to me. People greeted me as I stepped through. The opportunities were not knocking at the door, they were entering without permission. Considering how they gathered in great numbers, there was little I could do but send most of them away. I now had the opportunities which were once out of reach. As I placed my hands around each choice, I realised that it was an illusion. I had not changed. I had not chosen to change but, yet, my life had. People did not care how I had arrived. They were only interested in what I could do for them. I was successful. I was good to be around; I was wanted.

My parents now also seemed to want me. They would attend my choir performances and stand in line with other parents to receive the applause. My previous concerts had been delivered without applause; they were never attended. Now they waited to receive fame for my success. The change had also changed them.

***

But one thing which did not change was their generosity. No, it did. It got worse. When the materialistic holiday of Christmas had passed I found myself more deprived and feeling less loved.

How was I to interpret the economy-sized package of paper napkins my mother had wrapped as a gift? Or the bottle of home-made barbeque sauce which lay broken in a box and stinking up my Christmas? When she told me, "there's a little left," the insanity became clear. I'm happy to say, this time I was not alone. She mailed boxes of Wheaties to my cousins.

***

The relationship began to change me and continued to develop along with its own rituals. When the weekend would arrive, we would quickly pack our bags and run away. There would be no sin worse than staying in town and being caught in the act. The ritual became routine, slowly losing its meaning and becoming increasingly tiring. Why couldn't we step out into the night and live within the city in which we lived? But not even the darkness was safe enough to hide the crime that was undressing between us. Even when I was alone, I was fearful of being caught although I was not the criminal.

ALMOST NORMAL

But slowly my association with the doctor began to rub off on me. My actions became increasingly secretive, and the only words which my mouth could form were lies. As the lies slipped more easily across my lips, the pain of hiding the truth took over, and I bit into my lip to taste the blood which was becoming sour within me. I then told myself it was all right to continue the deceit; these were white lies. Once again I had lied, this time, to myself.

I took my lies, packed them into my book bag, and started attending an expensive, private college. As I moved through the hallways and started to attend my different classes, I began to learn to live another lie.

No one really wanted the truth anyway. I told everyone that my grandparents were supporting me; they seemed far enough away. I threw out my old raggy jean jacket, and replaced it with dress shirts and pants. I was rather convincing; as the hard face of reality was washed and pressed, I began to "look" like I belonged. And along with Belonging, arrived Acceptance; these visitors carried along with them not only more respect but better grades. These were other reasons for trying to "fit in" and be normal.

I took my illusion of normalcy with me down

town. One of my classes required that we break bread with the indigent, and be their servants. As I served, I wondered. Who were these people, and why were they living like this? They seemed like they were on the other side of town, miles away from school, but they were only a few minutes away. After serving them, I sat down with them to pick at the food I was required to eat. As I suspected, the food was not very good, and I would have preferred to throw it out. But as the teacher looked on, I forced myself to eat. I didn't want a taste of their food or their reality. They could consume it. It wasn't for me, I wasn't coming back.

So I went back to continue to live out my lie in a studio apartment a few miles away from the doctor. It was an address in which to send my package of deceit. But I was never there to receive it, I was always at his house, hiding, hoping no one would find me.

But he had found me, and he seemed the perfect man for me. He was well aware of the dark disturbing features of my character and had not been frightened enough to lock the door and leave me outside knocking. Although I had to hide from the rest of the world, I didn't have to hide from him - he knew everything. Because of this we grew close to one another rather quickly. So while the truth weakened, our lies became stronger.

ALMOST NORMAL

The many trips we took were close to home, empty and shallow. But one time we ventured out, wondering if the world further out would have more to offer. In Colorado Springs we stayed at the Broadmoor. It was an interesting experience. The few channels which informed me about the Broadmoor and what there was to do at the Broadmoor, did little to entertain my severe sunburn. As I lay in bed flipping meaningless channels, I would gaze at the only thing worth looking at - the beautiful view outside my window, outside my room. While I did this, he played golf. We then would meet for lunch in a room filled with octogenarians, and I would slowly chew my salad, waiting, certain that one of them would pass away at any moment. But nothing happened at the Broadmoor, and I was so bored that I thought I would pass away. But then I went for a ride that I will never forget.

In Colorado Springs I slid into my new Honda Accord, and parked the $500.00 oil leaking pile of metal I had driven for good. I was hysterical. I was now not only living in a new world, I was driving in it. There was no way I was going to slow down or put on the brakes to the life which was before me. I drove forward, back home, in my new car, carefully breaking it in. I loved the smell and the security of my new car. It was mine, all mine!

When I arrived home, I went further, to see my parents and to show them *my* car. They didn't have much to say, and they didn't seem to care. But I was amazed. Suddenly my good looks had extended far beyond me, reaching their destination before I did. My arrival was welcomed even before they knew who I was.

I was beginning to understand that with money it didn't matter who people thought I was. As long as he knew me, and wanted me, I could continue to move forward.

It was as I was moving forward that I was slightly taken aback by the appearance of his ex-wife. Pregnant by another man and lost, she moved in with my doctor. Because I had been found, I felt for her, and I agreed to be comfortable with this arrangement. She and the doctor were no longer in love but just friends. She didn't want to be with him, but she didn't want me to be with him either. I didn't realise she was doing everything in her power to separate us.

Unaware that the emotional distance was growing between us, I moved farther away to a nearby city to attend the state university. I thought that my education would cost less, and I would be less of a burden on him. Truly, I thought that I would be less dependent on him. But I ended up

ALMOST NORMAL

not only learning a lot, I paid a lot.

She soon followed, bringing along with her the undermining tricks she would play. We were not only attending the same school, we were in the same chemistry class. She experimented with my feelings convincing me that I was her friend - so I thought. At first, when I called for her she was there for me; I was always there for her. But as she spread her phoniness out into the campus, she attracted a few followers. She no longer needed me. Now I would call, but no call would ever be returned. Then out of the blue she came over to cry on the familiar shoulder reserved for her. But she was only there because she was lost and alone, with no one to turn to. It wouldn't have been so bad if she had just used me, but she would take the things I had said in confidence to her, stretch and twist them, and then return them to him.

***

To be less of a burden, I rented an apartment on the shadier side of town. I looked out my only window and decided that I had made a mistake when I rented this place. I told her that he would have to understand that the darkness was smothering me, and that I would have to find a better place.

Ann Kolsrud

She told him that I said that I was going to rent a penthouse apartment, and if he wouldn't go along with it, I was going to sue him.

***

At first, it was all right that she had altered the truth because I was always able to correct the things that had been warped. The doctor had always believed me. But with the increasing distance came an increase in mistrust. I interpreted this growing distance in the relationship as room to move, and I now accepted the opportunity to explore another relationship. But as I began to move in another direction so did my mind. As I moved within my freedom I found myself increasingly bound by my problems. By the fall semester I only ended up finishing two classes, but by the spring semester I had to withdraw from school.

***

She found herself, and I found myself lost. She had played many games, and lucky for her, she had good scores - she was admitted to medical school. I really don't understand why they even allow such little people to play? I'm sure she is still playing. Even after she becomes a doctor she will continue to hide her true nature and seek out people to use - this time her true

ALMOST NORMAL

nature will be hidden underneath a big white coat.

Chapter Nine

It was as if I was dreaming. I continued to check myself as she spoke; was I really here, was I truly hearing this? She sat next to me as these thoughts ran through my mind. She was a beautiful brunette. It wasn't just her physical attributes that attracted me to her, but also, her free confident spirit which seemed to emanate from her being. She talked about the music she liked, the books she had read, and any other profundity which seemed to pique her interest. The moment seemed ethereal and intangible; I wondered if I would remember it. But somewhere between the drone of niceties and rigmarole, I heard her say her name was Jennifer, or "Jen" for short.

We continued to talk. We had a lot of interests in common, and we were the same age. The smoke-filled darkness, the camouflage of the bar was there to slowly allow an adjustment to another's imperfections, was no longer important; we were ready to face each other's flaws. So we carried our conversations and our imperfections to a 24 hour restaurant - it was now 4am.

Some magical force had led me down to the bar. It seemed to be some kind of destiny thing. Jen told me about the dream she had experienced which reaffirmed my conviction of divine intervention. I dropped Jen off at her car and we both went home. But for the next week we talked for at least an hour every night on the phone. It was long distance; otherwise, we would have talked longer.

I figured the best way to tell the doctor of my latest experiences was just to come out. I told him straight out that I had started dating a woman. He was curious and asked a lot of questions; I answered very few. I figured it was none of his business. He had encouraged me to explore other relationships, and that was what I was doing. I still loved the doctor, but at this point I loved him as a parent, a mentor. I was committed now to Jen and he would have to understand that. I continued to date Jen, and I kept in touch with the doctor. But I couldn't go too far away from him. The leash was not very long, and I was still "healing."

Although I tried to remain loyal to Jen, I found not only the leash to be short but I also found it around my neck. So at his convenience I found the doctor at my door. There he was at the door; the man who had opened doors, and the man who was still supporting me. Without hesitation, I let him in my apartment. I began to think of Jen and her feelings. How would she feel if she knew about him? If I didn't tell her it would be OK because that relationship was over, or wasn't it? The next thing I knew, I was embraced in his arms with the layers of my dignity falling to the floor; it was the first frost and the leaves had fallen to the ground- I was naked.

So with the small amount of dignity which remained, I continued; he would come and then he would leave. I gathered my clothes and went to see Jen. It was so nice to talk to her, and so nice not to talk about certain things. I knew to be fair to her I really needed to be honest with her. But how could I? How could I tell her? I had been so evil: hiding behind the dark lies and still looking her straight in the face. I began to bloom in the shadows and fade in the sun; I was safe in the shadows of a lie and in danger if any light came to the now hidden truth. But I wasn't big enough to hold all the lies anymore, and so I allowed the truth to escape. I loved Jen; I needed him. But I ended up losing my love, and finding myself in great need.

***

Everyday is about the same now; little by little I slowly begin to decompensate, despite my attempts to grow. My thoughts are motionless, existing within a narrow spectrum of each day's events. I often find myself thinking of them. I drive the existing memories I have of them wherever I go; I am their chauffeur. It seems only yesterday that I had friends, money, respect, and happiness; in other words, I had a life.

I become very frightened in public when I see people who resemble my former friends. I don't know exactly why this is. I think part of my fear in seeing these people come from the truth - I am so humbled. I have slipped and have lost my confidence; the sickness has marched back into my life.

But the fact remains, no matter how much I think about them, I cannot bring them back. It is their grasp and touch which ultimately brings soothing to my troubled heart.

I remember Jen. I don't believe that I could find a person as intelligent and as sensitive as she was. Why I was so blind to this vision? I blame my lack of focus. I miss her.

Sometimes I drive by his former place of residence. I find myself covering the distance to his home. Things have changed; there is now a house at the dead-end near his house. So I park my car and stare at the changes which have occurred and that my mind fights to accept. It's hard to believe that this was once my neighbourhood - I fit in. Now I do not belong here. So I visit in fear, hoping that they do not think that I'm a criminal on the prowl.

Chapter Ten

After losing my love I was nowhere to be found, that is if anyone was looking. And with my newly found great need, I found myself lost with great loss. With a stinging slap to the face, reality had hit me; I now had to adjust from lounging in hotel rooms which were 500 dollars a night to struggling to live on 500 dollars a month. I was so out of place and wandering with no hope of being discovered. Now no one could find me and fill the void.

I began to move deeper into my sickness following the innate plan that would bring success to the heist. The only thief was the illness which now began to steal my thoughts and my entire personality. The person that had once belonged to me had been taken from my possession. Many reports were made and documented, but my property would forever remain unclaimed.

There were many days in which I would try to find myself. I would sit for hours on end staring at blank walls; smoking cigarettes and listening to the dispatch send unmarked cars to monitor me. The days became weeks, and my mouth filled with the slime from the loss of personal hygiene. All my energy now had to be directed at saving myself; placing myself on my own most wanted list. They would not leave me alone. As I attempted to leave them by switching channels, I only found that each channel contained its own talk show in which I was the focus of intense ridicule. Carefully I unplugged all the appliances; it was through this connection to the outside that they would try to reach me, and influence me. I covered the windows with tin foil to block out further radiation. Only at night did I dare to peek out the window and risk exposure. When I did look out, I looked out to a world so near to being away. Armageddon had begun. I sat shaking, fearful of personally confronting any arch angels.

I attempted to call my parents. Even though they were usually only a few miles away they now had been transported to the part of the universe which was slipping away. I talked quickly, trying to explain, and prepare them. But no matter how desperately I wanted to warn them, they could not understand me. The connection was fading.

Before the firing squad completed its sentence, I decided that for my final request I would have a drink. The next thing I knew was that a lot of people had found me. They told me that I was almost there, and I was. I was in an ambulance headed to the hospital to have my stomach pumped. I was in and out, never making any decision to stay. The doctor kept asking me if I had taken any other pills. I came in to tell him "no." Then to my surprise he said to the nurse that he had found some more. I went out again.

They filled me full of charcoal to absorb the overdose. I couldn't hold it in and I ended up shitting all over myself. I overheard them saying to make this a real bad experience for me so I wouldn't do it again. But I didn't understand. "I" hadn't done anything. At least I didn't *remember* doing anything.

I was now in and the doctor came over to talk to me. Because I didn't have my glasses on and I could not see, his words seemed even less clear to me. He told me that this was how Marilyn Monroe had died. Suddenly he made sense to me, for I was a movie star; I had been on every channel.

***

I was dreaming, and in my dream all the small little creatures climbed over and above me. I was left looking down at how low I was now and how far the distance between us had become. My guts wrenched in agony from this painful realisation; another nightmare of pure hell. I woke up with the relief that it had only been a dream. After realising that the dream was true; an accurate reflection of my life, I was filled with terror. Not even my dreams could be an escape

ALMOST NORMAL

for my painful reality.

***

I continued to try to find myself. I sat a lot, not moving in space or time, smoking heavily and staring at nothing that made sense. I began to drink a lot - for me. Since I was lost I let the people around me, direct me. They had convinced me that now I had become some kind of an alcoholic. Yes, I was mentally ill and I drank, so I must be an alcoholic - they thought. So I followed their directions to a nearby detox centre. There I was placed in the prison clothes in which I had always belonged, and treated as the inmate that had been sentenced from birth. Even though I was cold, they would not give me my jacket for fear of escape. They didn't realise that I really wasn't ever going anywhere. I watched the others shake as the poison left their bodies. The sounds of vomiting contributed to the disorder, and we only got in line when we were to eat. It was here that I realised that I had once again been misled. Although I had been abusing alcohol, I was not an alcoholic. With desperation, I begged to be paroled, and they approved. As I was leaving, they sent me off with a sarcastic, "See you later." Only I knew what was true. I would not see them later; I would not return to the stereotypical pigeon hole in which they had placed me.

Chapter Eleven

I had been gone awhile, and upon my return realised that I needed to find a new doctor. I tried to inconspicuously crawl back into treatment, but there were too many holes to fill besides the ones in my head. I walked into one office after another, running out, withdrawing from the conversations which probed deep into an area which I had silenced long ago.

Curiosity had killed more than the cat; it had begun to kill me. I was in desperate need of a doctor, but it was difficult to find one whom I didn't know, or rather, one who didn't know me. I was afraid. They were all so high above me that it would be easy for them to look down - and some did. It had been *me* that had crossed the line. I was responsible for corrupting the professional relationship. They needed to be careful of me for I was the dangerous one. But the truth is that I was more afraid of them. Together they could destroy me for coming so near to their law-suit fragile world. There would never be complete trust again, let alone respect. I had been damaged.

***

It's hard to see black writing on black paper, let alone, damage to a person who is already damaged. So I continue to write the words of my pain on the paper, although I know that they will never be read, and that only I will know them.

***

So I walked a plank, on a ship of trust. And there I remained, wondering if I would ever be made to jump. But I had found a doctor that allowed me to remain standing, and eventually I was able to walk on from there. Because of the distance I moved closer. I planted my feet, in low-income housing, across the hall from one of my few friends.

It was nice to be so close to a friend, since friends were so far and few between. We were together a lot, although we did very little. Eventually our hunger drove us out into the city, downtown; to the place I had thought I would never return. And as I stood in line with the other poor people, I noticed how my clothing stood out. Still fresh from my picking, it made me feel even more out of place. I hid my jewellery in my pockets, to make me look less misplaced; I did belong here. Although I noticed a few looks no one said a word. I lowered myself into a chair, and began to put the food into my mouth. I looked up suddenly to see if I could catch anyone looking at how out of place I was. But all I saw was a personal message from God himself: he was fucking with me.

The same class and the same teacher, with whom I had served the poor, were now serving me. I saw the teacher, and I wondered if I was even too low to crawl over and talk with her. But I wanted to know. So I made my way through the maze of people to speak with her. After seeing that she remembered me, I told her of my situation. Then I asked, "Did you ever suspect that I was different?"

"No" she said. "I just remember you as a person who asked a lot of questions."

I had not been back for three years. Four days out of the week they served the poor. Each day, a different organization sponsored the dinner, and yet my fate had allowed me to return to taste while the life I had before, served. So after experiencing something beyond coincidence, I went home full. Although I felt very sick to my stomach, I now knew that there had to be a reason for my life. So my friend and I returned home together, but she went to sleep, and I continued with my purpose.

Cindy was one of us. Although I didn't understand her problems I understood her struggle, and she mine. So when the day came that the pain tried to go, I found myself frozen with confusion. There she lay on the bed, suffocating the overdose she had taken with a plastic bag. I didn't know what to do. The world was really not such a great place, and I "loved her enough to let her go." But I called for help - help to help me make a decision and help to help her, to save her from dying.

We had both survived, only to risk our lives by living within halls blood-smeared from occasional stabbings. My fear was so great that I blocked the door with a chair and table every night.

One night a man kept retracing the steps that led to my door. I had taken my medicine, and was slowly drifting off into a fog as I became curiously afraid. When I looked under the door to see that his feet were gone, I opened the door to see if he had finally left me alone. Suddenly I could smell his breath as he pushed his way into my apartment. The fear seized my breath, and I slammed the door shut so I could breathe. I woke up the next morning, looking under my pillow for any signs of the truth. But it is still an unknown, and I still live in fear that I was unknowingly raped. I could not force upon myself the belief that I was not a victim
.

While living in fear, one day, I sat alone aware of the subtle smell of the gas stove. If fact, the whole building smelled of the cooking appliance. Suddenly, I became aware of a phone ringing down the scary hall. It would not stop. There was no one to answer it except the gas which had accumulated. They were trying to blow up the building! My fear called the landlord, but I only told him that the phone would not stop ringing.

Then one day I dared to peek out, and down the long, treacherous hall, I saw a figure. All was quiet, and there it lay. I wondered if it was really there. I approached cautiously. I wasn't sure if it was living or dead and I didn't want to get too close. So I walked back to my apartment and called 911. I watched them arrive and then I closed the door; this time I didn't want to know.

ALMOST NORMAL

Chapter Twelve

It was at this time that I put closure to the possibility of opening the doors to my parents. If they loved me, why didn't they rescue me? Did I mean so little that they would allow me to slip away, out of their hands, to dangle in front of the vicious teeth of the world which was vying to erase me. I hung precariously with the fangs only inches away preparing to rip me from any sense of security and well being. Surely they would come look me up, or perhaps call me. But their calls reflected their love for me: distant and indirect. I would call collect, they would deny me, and call me back at their leisure. Before they had signed a release, I was gone. I had been removed from my home to the intestines of society to be dissolved among the other trash.

The experience was painful, and they were too far away to hear my small, struggling voice. If I became angry, they became angrier at me - for being born. I screamed to be loved, and to feel the touch which had welcomed me into this world. Where was it now, when I needed it most? I prayed for my parents to reclaim me, but every small hope which dared to peek out from under was smothered. Without parents, I soon gave up. I began to pray to God to reclaim me, for he was my only father.

Chapter Thirteen

I didn't like taking pills. I always questioned if they had been tampered with, or perhaps were just placebos. Worse yet, I feared the disease-like illnesses which ravaged my body in the form of side-effects. But the mental pain was great enough that I swallowed my doubt and fear, along with the pills and made myself believe. If I could do anything to ease this struggle within my faith, I would. But it was a philosophy built on a precarious foundation. Did the positive attributes of the medicines out-weigh the negative effects? It didn't matter; I had learned to follow blindly. So regardless of how I felt about the medicines, I took them as prescribed. But because I carried the mark of mental illness everywhere I went, few people held little faith in me. Not only was I incapable of taking medicine correctly, a cloud of potential drug abuse hung intertwined with the cloud of stigma. When the physical pain also became great enough, they ex-communicated me from the care found within their community, and sent me away to find my own salvation.

Fewer pills meant a smaller struggle, so in turn, I decided to discontinue my birth control pills. But the struggle only grew bigger; suddenly, I had pain like never before. Curled up with a bottle of ibuprofen, I said a few prayers begging that the few pills I could take would safely remove the pain from my womb. But I knew the pain would not leave even if I tried to kill it with an entire bottle. So I reached out connecting myself to a pharmacist, and the hope that there was something which could be prescribed to ease the pain. Growing faint, I reached out one more time to call my gynaecologist. Then with a quick slice into my hope, the connection was severed; They told me "no" they couldn't help me. So with the little life which remained within me, I decided that I would have to go back on birth control; it was one more pill, but it provided a smaller struggle.

Then it happened I was all alone, facing the potential impregnation of pain, with no one to believe me, or even understand; I was on my own. Although I was in the hospital again, there was no one to help me. The struggle would soon return, so I insisted that they provide the support I needed and give me my birth control. They asked for the name of my gynaecologist and assured me that I would not be alone. But the delivery of the message had been difficult, and things went wrong. The staff then handed me a phone, and on another end was the approval for which I was waiting so that I could take the birth control pills. Somewhere along the way, in my attempts to connect, they had gotten lost; they thought the pills had caused me the pain. I began to get upset thinking of the intense labour I was now experiencing and how it would continue to grow within me. With desperation, I explained that they were lost; I had found that I desperately needed the pills. But no matter how I tried, they could not understand me. I laid down the phone of one-way conversation and headed to my room crying. With the ringing of yet another phone, I had found myself, this time, with tears.

***

It doesn't matter that the bed in which you lay is in an expensive hotel. The guests ignore you, that is, if they can even see you. And when you call for the bell boy, you better hope that you know his language, or perhaps, he will just turn around and leave.

ALMOST NORMAL

Chapter Fourteen

One day I woke up and it dawned on me that the shadows in my life had touched me in private places. They had not only left their mark they had infected me with a horror that would possibly out-live me. It was this day that I decided to pull the plug on my fertility.

I knew with the "right" man, my children would be fashion models, so incredibly beautiful and intelligent. But I also knew that with the "right" man my children would be almost guaranteed to follow my endless road of torture. With any man, the risk was too great. So, to protect others, I closed my road to unpredictable danger, and scheduled myself to be repaired, and sterilized - a tubal ligation.

I told the doctor to fix me good, and remove the possibility of the infection from spreading; I wanted no chance of pregnancy. Because of the operation not only did I have an end to my fertility, I had a name for the pain which had previously impregnated me; I was diagnosed with endometriosis. I gave little thought or attention to my new diagnosis, distracted by the emptiness which had crawled into me.

There were many reasons for arriving at this decision. If I could not care for myself, no matter how much I wanted to care, I could not care for another person. I knew that I wouldn't have any help. My parents told me long ago, that they were finished raising a child; although I wonder when they had started. It had been an easy decision, but it had not been an easy action. The removal of my fertility was just one more strike against my feelings of normalcy. Not only would I be a little more alone in life, I would once again be a little more abnormal.

My friends have kids, my cousins have kids, and almost everyone it seems has kids. So, I act as if I couldn't care less, as if kids are just an irritating wound that lasts a long time. When they say to me, "Would you like to hold the baby?" I quickly, coldly decline. If they only knew that these children each time reopen a wound for me that will never heal. I cry for my children whom I never gave a chance to enter into the world. But I find comfort in knowing that I have probably saved them from a life of tears.

So now every time I have a female problem, and I call to speak to a nurse, they ask if I am pregnant. Not only does the wound reopen but I am reminded that I am a little less needed and a little more alone in life.

***

ALMOST NORMAL

I have a baby, although no one recognises this. No one helps me pay his bills, or appreciates the responsibility involved. They also do not understand that I love him like my own. When mother's day arrives, rarely does anyone acknowledge my position. But my dog loves me and that is all that matters - besides now I am successful!

Chapter Fifteen

I wanted to be normal. I would have sold my soul to have what others seemed to have, but instead I just risked my life. So they put me on a medicine which while promising to bring back my life, could take it away - forever. Every week I had to go have a blood test to make certain that forever would never come. But it didn't, and I seemed to improve almost instantly. I began to taste not only some of the stability I had lost long ago, but also everything in sight. With the benefits, I paid a heavy price - 80 lbs or so. There was nothing I could do. The helplessness which had been taught to me, I had now learned. So while being accepted as more normal, I was rejected in a new way - I was fat.

I was now overweight with an explanation for my condition. But an explanation would only bring more questions, and I had to remain quiet. So with every thundering step, a storm of disgust began to brew within me. It was this burden I had to carry which only added to the weight.

But I was more normal, wasn't I? Every day, I had smoked four packs of cigarettes. And then one day I just stopped. My parents praised me greatly for this accomplishment. But how can you accomplish something which had required basically no effort?

ALMOST NORMAL

Anyway, I appeared to be on some road back. I began by walking; delivering the local paper to my neighbourhood.

Because I had been so lost and feeling that I couldn't follow a map on my own, someone went with me the first few times. I was always worried that a paper would get lost in some pot hole of my unpaved memory. I panicked that at the end I would be short, and my job would be unfinished. Eventually I knew my way, and I moved on to a more demanding job; I had found my route.

Through supported employment, I pursued a new opportunity. While internally nervous, I confidently captured each question of the interview and was hired. But someone didn't like me, and drove miles out of her way to drop me in a pool of sharks.

With each complaint I became panicked and found myself breathless in fear of the next attack. But no matter how many times the sharks came around the wounds were never serious enough to fire me, only serious enough to kill me. The other people whom I worked with told me to relax, that this girl had no power. But despite these reassurances from others, I knew she was more dangerous to me than they could ever know; the stress was beginning to devour me.

Six months later, I removed myself from the pool of harassment which had surrounded me. The supervisor felt bad about the situation, and my co-worker insisted that I list my reason for leaving as the constant harassment which I had to endure. With this added stress, my illness had begun to surface and had begun to pull me down deep where there was no oxygen. The only thing keeping me afloat was me. Meanwhile, the so-called support I was receiving was just a net full of holes. They told me that I hadn't given the job a chance or them. But I did give them a chance. I gave them a chance to understand that I had been harassed. Although everyone at work knew this and my co-worker had shared this with my job coach, I fell through their net of holes to become entangled in their disbelief. As they continued to hold me underwater, I could vaguely see the skeletal remains of the truth they had discarded which could set me free.

***

People often believe that normal things cannot happen to abnormal people. If I have pain, it's in my head. If I am attacked, I am being paranoid. And if I am being harassed, I am just "letting every little thing get to me." It doesn't matter that I have normal people to prove these things. Some people have already convicted me;

guilty before proven innocent - with no trial. So, I carry my conviction that I was innocent, but I have lost every appeal.

Eventually I dropped my campaign for justice knowing that I would never win. They had won, hands down, but I will always remain bitter knowing that I am the better candidate.

***

I moved on without the support I had never really had and got another job - on my own. This time I was not only eating food, I was selling it. I had been offered the opportunity to interview for the job. After a successful interview, the apple itself was offered - and I bit. Although I barely imagine being able to hold it in my sickly grasp, I held my breath taking one day at a time until the bright colour of its newness began to fade along with my insecurity. I had achieved it, I had conceived it, and although very little, I could imagine it. I continued to be amazed with what I was able to do; I had never been this close to normal.

Chapter Sixteen

Because I was now so close to being normal, I thought perhaps I was not only close, I had already arrived. Maybe I really didn't need the medicine. There had been a place before in my life where I didn't really need medicine, a rest stop along an old tiring highway, with a destination that could never be reached. Hoping for a good rest, I went off the medicine, but ended up having a very bad trip.

Almost immediately I began to get sick - physically. I wasn't sure where I was or in which direction I was headed. Sometimes I went straight north and suddenly finding myself chilled to the bone. The next minute, I was headed south and melting. I was up and down to remove the sweat soaked blankets which covered my sick body. Then my intestines started down a windy road of their own, leaving me, many times, stranded in the bathroom. For two weeks, I continued to travel through this physical hell. Along the way, hives began to pop up and cover my body to form a topographical map of their own. Eventually I returned to work. But for every mile the physical illness retired, the mental illness actively pursued.

Now I could not sleep. At first I was lucky if I could get 3 hours of rest. I was feeling bad about the work I had already missed, so I made myself go back anyhow. I would arise in the morning from my short sleep to the violent awakening of my intestines. I learned not to eat and to take a lot of Imodium. This seemed to dampen the physical part, but the fire in my head seemed to burn out of control. My sleep was getting worse.

I went to work - this time, a real zombie. I already had a lot of challenges waiting for me when I arrived at work. Every time I was fearful that I had given the wrong change back, and many times I would ask the customer if I could count it again. So I would count it again and hand it back to the customer often never fully releasing it.

My compulsiveness was obvious, and I did everything in my power to make light of it and hide the ferocious obssessiveness. But now that sleep had walked out of my life, the struggle to handle my symptoms had walked all over me. I kept moving - it hurt to stand. Things continued to worsen. My feet and hands were now swollen from my hives, and I was so tired, I was sick. I was actually afraid that I could become cataplectic. I was quickly fading on my feet. Then there was a knock at my door. I opened it only to face an irate customer who proceeded to slap me. All the pain was so great that I almost passed out. Then the pain increased even more; I had become aware that I could no longer do my job. I would have to miss more work. Then the bagger leaned over and said to me that she had wanted to call in sick because she had a Spanish test.

***

I have a hard time believing someone when they tell me that they are "depressed" because they missed a movie. And if they haven't slept for one night, I wonder if they truly know what "tired" is. While I wouldn't wish the real thing on anyone, I sometimes wish that they at least understood. So while I gain the meaning of some words and stretch the meaning of others, I wonder if I am truly "loved."

ALMOST NORMAL

Chapter Seventeen

The sleep that I increasingly desired became more distant - a dream in itself. My psychiatrist began to prescribe sleeping medication. This medication which I was told would knock out a normal person for 24 hours was able to provide me 3. But these few hours were only a nightmare.

The nightmare would begin as every small sound hit me with a blast, throwing me violently into a panic. When I could drift off, I was sometimes sucked under. There would be dreams in which I had become even more lost. In these dreams, I would wake up not knowing where I was and unable to ask the people around me. As I endured the torture of a mind lost and confused, they would carry me away kicking and screaming. The nightmare would then proceed as I woke up to find myself caught in this hell unable to escape. So, I would hit myself, until the (I hoped) real world would connect with my brain.

As I grew increasingly tired, I grew increasingly weary. Was life worth living? There was no reason to go back on such a dangerous medicine just because I couldn't sleep. So my doctor added another sleeping medicine on top of the one I was already taking. He promised me that this combination would make me sleep. But I was becoming doubtful. I told him that if this did not work, I had to be put in the hospital. I did not know that I would go on even longer.

As I expected, the additional medicine did not change a thing - it was worthless. I continued to hope that sleep would reclaim me, so I postponed the inevitable - starting the meds again. Then one morning I ended up in the emergency room. The hives had consumed my body while I hung helpless at the end of my rope. The ER doctor gave me the usual shot - epinephrine, or a taper of steroids. I climbed back in control able to mention the unbearable insomnia. Suddenly he grew irritated and told me that he was **not** going to start treating a sleeping problem at 7:30 in the morning. I left with the rope tightening around my neck.

I spoke to my doctor's nurse. They had failed to help me, and I could no longer continue to try. With their blessing, my mother drove me 2 hours away to the state university's emergency room.

I now spoke to a doctor. I explained that I needed help to sleep. Perhaps special monitoring or whatever the marvel of modern medicine could offer. I thought I needed to be in the hospital. But they wouldn't admit me. They wouldn't even call my doctor - they didn't want to bother him. I was told that they do not admit people just because they can't sleep, and since I wasn't having symptoms - yet. But then I suddenly grew too tired to exist, and I began to lose my mind. Tears began to stream down my face. I tried to hold them back, but I was too tired. The doctors came back to ask me what was going on - was I suicidal? Being too proud to lower myself to threats of suicide just to get help, I said "no."

They sent the remaining part of me home with a bottle of the medicine which had somewhat helped, and told me to call my doctor in a few days.

As my mother drove me home, my pride balanced precariously on a tight-rope of existence. When I arrived home, I took the plunge and consumed the whole bottle. I didn't want to kill myself, but I was so tired I wanted to die. I grabbed the phone and described my final attempt at sleeping to someone. The ambulance arrived, and this time, they admitted me to the hospital.

The medication had been liquid, so they really couldn't pump my stomach. I had been saved from reliving my experience from the past. But how saved was I really? That night I didn't sleep at all.

***

Ann Kolsrud

The first night of insomnia, is a tiring re-run which everyone sees at some point in their life. When the unending exhaustion spreads to a week it becomes a cult classic B movie. But when, after a month, you find yourself somehow still moving you know that you are witnessing pure evil.

I try desperately to close my eyes to the violence but a bright light continues to shine on the back of my mind, producing these images. When I complain they ask if I have tried drinking warm milk. Then they go home to sleep, and I stay up to watch another movie.

ALMOST NORMAL

Chapter Eighteen

As I had declined physically, I had eroded mentally, and the flood which ensued had destroyed any hopes of reclaiming any land on which to rest. So I eagerly consumed my medication again.

Soon things were close to normal again. My ability to work returned to me, and it seemed my possibility of a future had also returned; so I went back - to school.

While working, I laboured to pick up the pieces dropped years ago. I took Biology 2 and Chemistry 2, trying to begin to understand the science of which I was a product - I got A's. I continued to learn although I discovered to my disappointment, some questions would never be answered.

Chapter Nineteen

When the spring semester had ended, I fell back to a slower pace. It was at this time that my doctor came forward with the idea of adding a new medication to the one I was already taking. He had heard that if I were to combine the past with the present, I could have a better future. The new medication possibly could suppress my insatiable appetite; the long awaited rescue from my island of hunger within the seas of salivation. It was worth a try. Summer would be a good time to explore. I would quickly claim the future and return to the present to continue with school. The future was better, and I thought it would be even better if I could get rid of the past completely. Newer was better, wasn't it? So my doctor took me off the medication I had taken for almost five years and switched me completely to the new one.

It wasn't just that I thought that the new medicine would be better. I didn't enjoy the weekly blood draws. It wasn't the physical pain which I wanted to avoid but the mental pain. I thought perhaps that they would stick me with a dirty needle - with or without intention. Or worse, people would think I was a junkie - for I already had track marks; from the many miles the razor blades had travelled.

I had great faith in the new medicine; its

touch would heal me. It was a miracle; I was cured. My belief in the old medicine became lost when I realized its deception; despite my success it had not only made me fat, but also lazy. Suddenly, I had been moved, not only to succeed, but to take care of myself. The emotions which had been so suppressed began to emerge. Now not only could I have success, I could feel it. And even without, I could have happiness. I had returned. Now, not only had I reclaimed a part of how I had felt before becoming ill, I could smell it. In fact I could smell so much that I had to quit breathing when I passed through the meat department of our local store. I began to wonder if my heightened sense of smell was normal. I decided that I would prefer to have any sense of smell than none.

***

I remember a better time when my rotting body had vitality, and the days were filled with the smell of excitement. Although I moved back into my apartment three years ago, I have not been back since recently. As I regain the smell of the life lost, the memories come flooding back. Hungering to be where I once was, I can almost fool myself thinking that nothing has changed. But as each day slowly attaches new meaning to each smell, I am reminded that the past is long gone.

***

Everything was going as planned. This time, I was attending school full-time. My mind was spontaneous, jumping to catch any concepts which passed by me. It seemed that there was nothing with which I could not connect; there was no place, no time, or universe which I could not master.

Then I became weary. The creeping malaise which had begun to creep into my life, took hold, and strangled me. The bed itself seemed to have glued me to its surface. I struggled to move and carry my weight through my daily routine. If I dropped something, I cried because I knew I did not have the strength to pick it up. Something was very wrong. So I loaded up my dead-weight into a car and drove myself to the doctor to be pronounced dead. But there was nothing wrong; I was only having side-effects.

The doctor suggested that I find a different psychiatrist. The psychiatrist I had been seeing was good - when I needed a prescription. But he was not only bad, but completely worthless to me if I required anything more than a signature. And so from here, I began my journey to an end.

ALMOST NORMAL

Chapter Twenty

Along the way I stopped at the other psychiatrist in town but decided to move on. Although I was still moving, I had nowhere to go. In order to go out of town, I had to prove my needs were not being met here. But my needs were now and some later rendezvous would be too late. So while my intentions to find a new psychiatrist were packed away in a suit case by the door, my body lay in bed cursed with side-effects.

It seemed that now I was extra sensitive to touch. With every pin that pierced my skin, I grew increasingly mad. My beaten body became very bruised, and my heart pounded stakes into my chest. I began to have chest pain. But there was nothing wrong again - the EKG had been fine. It didn't matter that I had been diagnosed previously with cardiomyopathy - heart failure. I was starting to become mental; that's all it was, so why even check it out? But I pursued. I went out the door glancing at the suitcase which waited. Meanwhile I ran around in circles going nowhere with a list of physical complaints that had no end. My mind no longer connected to lessons or even the print on the paper; it was becoming impossible to read. I would dive down to the test which rested at the bottom of the deep end of the pool. But before I could capture any meaning, I found myself running out of air, and I would have to resurface. I continued to dive but it was no use, time had run out. I was getting C's; it was a sign to me that I was in trouble.

I went home and didn't go back to school. The suitcase still sat by the doorway - never moved. The tinfoil went up and the channels on TV began to capture my attention. I didn't know who to follow; the signs from the TV, or the signs I recognised as a clear picture that my illness was being broadcast.

But what really wore me down were the little infections nipping at the raw flesh of previous irritations, and the constant pain creeping in my bones. Suddenly, I had four infections at the same time. So I ran to three different doctors to clear them up. As I tried to rest and keep what remained of my sanity while these infections had infested my body, I was prescribed an anti-biotic which made me wretch. After a day of not being able to eat or drink, on top of the exhaustion from running around fighting infections and the pain which was now radiating down my legs, my sanity began to wear thin. As the frustration continued, what remained of my sanity began to show holes. Then my tongue died; the antibiotics they had given me gave me a yeast infection in my mouth. And with the death to my tongue, I could feel the death to my sanity crawling over me.

ALMOST NORMAL

Finally, after a long unwelcome stay the infections left - owing me; they had cost me a lot. My spirit now hung loosely on my bones holding on to the pain which had locked itself inside me. As my pain's demands for attention grew more demonstrative, the struggle to the medicine cabinet became increasingly arduous. Eventually all I could do was crawl into the backseat of the car and be driven to the hospital. Then, after the gestation of pain for over a month, I gave birth to its baby.

I was in labour many hours, and when it was over there was nothing to hold except fear that the pain would return. The endometriosis I had been diagnosed with a year ago had come alive. The pain that had been neglected in the past because people thought it was in my head, now received attention. I had a doctor who could look through the cloud of stigma in which others remained mesmerized. I now had the pills to pamper the pain and smother the fear.

***

I now held the only piece of sanity I could own tightly in my fist. I opened my hand up to see if it was still there and it disappeared. Despite the calm which had settled within me, I had cracked. I drove through town knowing I was not real, and that I was so close to non-existent that I might as well pull the trigger. I came home to die, but my fucking insanity kept me alive; if I died, who would take my dog out to go the bathroom?

So instead I called my parents so I could scream at them for all the injustice in my world. I didn't care what they thought; I didn't care what I made them think. Well, whatever I said made them come to me for Christmas.

They drove many miles to be with me, and then they drove me madder when they told me that they had given away all our family's precious Christmas heirlooms. They told me since I didn't "care" about Christmas they gave away the few touches of normalcy which had decorated our Christmas trees. I just began to cry. Then they became mad at me for "caring" so much.

***

One day I stopped moving in circles; I had found an end to my list, and I had a referral. I picked up the suitcase, and headed out of town.

ALMOST NORMAL

Chapter Twenty-one

I was on my way, but when I arrived I discovered that along the way I had lost something. The intentions which had for so long been carefully packed and patiently waiting had been stolen. They had been replaced. Now I found my soul lining the walls of my empty suitcase. There was little I could do but close it once again and keep moving. But I could not escape the feeling that I had been, somehow, violated.

It had taken so much effort to get where I was now at that I started to wonder if it had been really worth it. What more could they do for me? I was wanderlust.

The new was not as good as the old. Or at least I wasn't as functional. I crept quietly around town avoiding conflict, in fear that even a stare could ignite my ticking bomb. I ran out of buildings which threatened to blow up because of me. There was no escape, and I wished for no escape. I welcomed the possibility of being buried in the rubble, so far down that even the search dogs could not rescue me. But I continued tirelessly to keep my thoughts straight, and to avoid the ones which sent my car careening into a retaining wall.

I knew I couldn't exist like this; it was a

matter of time. So when I was offered an additional medicine that I hadn't tried, I saw no alternative other than to try. Once again the possibility of gaining weight weighed heavy on my mind. But anyway, fearfully optimistic, I began to take it. It didn't take long and soon the fear shrouded the optimism, and under a great veil, I began to hide.

This other medicine had made me ravenous. And while one appetite increased, my appetite for hope had been lost. My options were not limited, there were none. For every benefit there was a sacrifice; every medicine affecting me differently, and bringing out a different person. I wondered who "I" really was.

***

I can be a fat slob counting change for others while I remain short-changed in my life. Or I can be frail and weak, as I attempt to push myself forward with the enormous weight of the illness in front of me. When the illness rules, I will sacrifice anything to escape its dictatorship. But after its strength has been suppressed by the medications, I will do anything to escape the weight quickly accumulating from the medications side-effects. It is very difficult to figure out which escape actually saves me. Quite often I make a decision and find my mind changed.

ALMOST NORMAL

At times I find myself wandering in an empty field, searching for words I once used to communicate. And as I count the blades of grass in this empty field I realise that I find myself enjoying intricate Calculus problems. Then suddenly without warning, the blades of grass become flowers: beautiful words which are picked from my choosing. I now can articulate but am unable to add the words in each sentence. I never know which way I will be. However I do know that in some way, I am both.

***

I was tired of trying to be outside of myself. It was much easier and safer being with myself than sorting through conversations with many different messages, movements on a face, alone, adding deception or clarity. And with the realisation that my symptoms would continue to weigh on me and things would not get easier, I dared to one more time risk my life. So I returned to the past; to receive the present, and the required blood draws. I was poked by needles and prodded by my self-esteem; in two months I had gained back over fifteen pounds. I wondered which was worse: to be rejected for what people can't see, or to be rejected for what people can see? Then I looked at myself in the mirror; there I stood reflecting at the terror I knew was within and gazing at the mountain which could not escape my window.

Although I stood so high, I felt so low. My beauty remained, but because of the mass which now surrounded it, its clarity had faded. As I looked on straining to see a memory, I realised it wasn't worth it. To remember, not only how I had been but how I had looked, were thorns. And so I prayed to Jesus to please remove them from my bleeding eyes.

The medicine which had brought me close to fitting into society, now, left me wandering in fields of sheep - but alone. As I tried to move back into society, I sat by a tree, watching them. I would protect them from me. This time the medicine had not worked. From here, there would be no return, and I would always somewhat regret that I had even left.

ALMOST NORMAL

Chapter Twenty-two

As I hid under my veil, I went out and got a job. Perhaps I wasn't ready, but when would I be? The medicine had not worked this time and there was nothing else. Pressure was mounting; you're not normal if you don't have a job, at least have a *real* excuse. So once again I pursued the empty net of support of supportive employment, and got a job packaging dog treats.

As I walked into the warehouse, I lifted my veil only to show a smile with no impetus. The place was crawling with lepers, or rather, other challenged people. With each carefully placed step, I feared contamination. As I breathed deeply to remove the air of exposure, I would be overrun with panic that a violent, horrible disease had walked over me. But I wanted to be normal, so I remained frozen, tortured within, as I placed dog biscuits in a box.

***

I wonder if anyone would take serious my fear of germs if they knew that I could die from it. In fact it is very serious - a very serious hypocrisy.

As I stand shaking in fear that I have

"caught" something, the torture from my fear is so consuming that I consider killing myself. I know that I am going to die from these germs and so my fate is certain. But as the panic swallows my breath and I struggle to breath, I try to save myself by reminding myself that I have wanted to die anyway. So why care if I have "caught" that final germ.

***

Then as I stood minding myself, the other criminals in the place began to riot. All they demanded is that they could exist as animals; vying for whatever they could. So as hair flew and piercing shrills disturbed the tranquillity, I ran within myself to find shelter. Although I was not the target, I had been hit. The experience skinned me alive. So although no one sees it, I lie on the floor as a decoration, a victim of trying to fit into society. So after the rampage had finally passed over me, I used my remaining life to call my employer and inform him that I would not be returning. Little did I know that any normalcy had died.

***

I have a pretty good idea when I'm eventually not going to make it into work; when I sit on the couch, paralysed by the hands of the

ALMOST NORMAL

clock, I know. I don't understand but no matter how much time there is, there is not enough time to move. "Soon" I will have to leave for work.

So as I fill with panic as the minutes tick away, I try to muster enough strength to re-teach my limbs how to get up and move. But with each attempt the memory only grows deeper until I reach the point where I can no longer go. So I make a phone call, write my letter of resignation and seal away in an envelope another failed attempt.

Chapter Twenty-three

After I quit working, I became very busy. The voices which had followed me throughout much of my life came knocking. Because they had become my friends, and they were the only ones who were consistently there for me, without hesitation, I let them in. Soon my hours were filled with supplying them with answers. We seemed so much as one that I wondered where they ended, and I started. Eventually, just as often as friends do, they grew distant. Soon they trailed behind me, following me everywhere I went, but staying far enough behind to point fingers. I prayed for release from their taunting, and it seemed as if God had answered my prayers. But instead of being released from their grasp, they had captured me. I no longer knew that I was even listening. Now as they directed me, I followed. Down to hell I would travel pursuing the words which were directed to kill me. Occasionally I would emerge from my great depths, but unable to realise where I had been, and what had happened.

***

I have forever, all my life, lived in fear of sharing the truth about the existence of voices, in fear that their exposure to the external world would send me to hell. But while the truth has remained somewhat buried, I have never been spared from being sent to hell. I suppose this is a revelation for me.

So while the demons continue to nail me to my own cross, I find relief in imagining a bullet shattering my skull, and killing me before they take my choice away and do it anyhow. Otherwise there is no way to run away from them.

I move through each day, trying to bring forward what I am able, and holding back the world within. Often the strain pulls so tight that I feel my forehead crack. Occasionally a word or sigh escapes, and someone near me will ask, "What?"

"Oh nothing," I answer.

I try to move past these directions by attempting to stubbornly pursue my own thoughts. But it is so exhausting moving against these currents. As I reach for a razor blade, I hope that the flow within my veins will appease the flow which attempts to overtake me. Then a loved one floats by on a raft to unknowingly rescue me. But sometimes their emotions (good or bad) upset me, and I jump back in to the water, still clinging to the raft for dear life. If I stand still in silence, sometimes there is an escape, and things aren't bad. But if I must move, the flood of voices returns drowning me while I breathe. So tonight I die, and wait for tomorrow to bring another death, always wondering when it will really end.

***

Although all I had wanted to do was crawl into a shell in which I fit, I was forced to continue outside, exposed and vulnerable. My Grandmother had become sick and there was no one else to help. So as I became emaciated from my insides being exposed to the outside, *she* kept me moving, pulling my ravaged carcass through the routine of social interaction. As I focused on the treacherous roads leading to my Grandmother's doctor appointment, *she* entertained. The more I watched as *she* remained so untrue to the feelings within, the more I grew to loathe her. So as *she* smiled, and talked to the doctor in charge of my grandmother's care, I imagined the sigh of relief that would follow after a bullet had entered my brain, releasing the strain between the two worlds. But *she* kept moving, like an automaton; an emptiness void of purpose, with hooks which snagged the fabric of this day's demands. I continued to hope for release, but *she* kept pulling me along - with her.

Then my grandmother suffering from the pain of aging, aged a little more from the pain. She then told me that she wanted God to take her. Why she wondered, had her prayers remained unanswered? I didn't know, but I did understand. My prayers also, had not been answered. So as the nurse tried to tell me that these feelings were expected in the elderly and understandably accepted, I wondered why my feelings weren't.

She continued until my grandmother was safe at home. Although my grandmother's prayers had not been answered, a few of mine had. *She* had released me. I crawled into my shell of safety, only to become dangerously lost within. Even if I were to place my body on another living thing, there would have been no contact. There was neither feeling to pass on nor any to receive. I had become another inanimate object with which to fill my house.

Not only had my mind shattered, the whole world had also. Everywhere I looked was a universe so connected, and at the same time so apart. Although I tried to close my eyes to the paradox before me, I could not close my ears. Although I resisted seeing the connection between the exhaust of a car, and the person attempting to speak to me, I was ordered to pay attention. Realising there was no way in which to blind myself from these tormenting displays of connection, I fell further apart.

I then was gathered together and shipped to my final appointment. I fought to move, as I felt myself becoming permanently fixed in position - with wings spread ready to fly. My voice had already given up; it was the thing I had to sacrifice just to keep moving. The only words worth struggling to bring forth, were the only words which could keep me out of the hospital. But as I strained to speak, their sound failed, and I was admitted.

ALMOST NORMAL

Chapter Twenty-four

Fucking pieces... Fucking torture... No escape.

***

I couldn't escape my imagination. I felt my wings spread, preparing for flight into a place I had never been. Only fear was my resistance to the apparent ease with which I could take flight. Fearing everyone would watch as I left, and that I could never return, I lowered my wings determined to fight to remain grounded. Such a fight took so much effort, and in order to make the competing sides fair, I remained quiet with no voice. The staff encouraged me to speak so that they could help me, but little did they know that my silence was not only helping me, it was saving me.

So I lay in my bed saving myself. I looked up at the light which prayed over me. In its reflection I saw myself. I laid my arms to my sides to form the cross of which I carried. With my pain, I was crucified, and I moved closer to Jesus. His hands and mine were one.

I existed as one with a room to myself. Outside many passed by. I listened as they spoke lies about me and attempted to apply damaging words to weaken my side of the ensuing battle.

Then a different voice passed outside my door. I gathered what little life I had within me I overheard another patient talks of sterilization - his fear of germs. After hearing his words my mind became infested with thoughts of disease. And as I grew concerned that a horrible disease would close the doors to my chance of being victor, I had become the victim. Some other door then closed, and I knew it was all signs from God that I had been contaminated and was now contagious. Why else would I be alone in my room?

***

I remember when I was a little girl and I spent the entire summer locked-up in my mind, inside the house. It was too dangerous to go outside; there were too many germs.

I would sit looking out a window watching all the other kids play. The fear was so great that I didn't even wish that I could be outside playing.

My father would come home from work, bringing with him the outside. Although I desperately wanted to give him a hug, I could not release the fear which I was already embracing. By some miracle, enough fear was washed away so I that I could leave the house. However, I was still isolated.

ALMOST NORMAL

***

Darkness had swallowed more than the day, but the light which followed was only from another morning. Much time had passed silently, although only to those on the outside. Inside there was no time and the battle raged on. I knew by the pain in my bladder that it could no longer remain inside. No matter how I tried to win the war over my body, I could not do it. With the battle to release such pressure lost, I returned to bed in pain and defeated.

Slowly with more time a small awakening occurred. As I dared to lift one eyelid, I looked towards the door - my way out. I was so shaken with the fear that one step outside would cover me with voices which were meaner, and which would deafen me with their screaming. But I was determined to get out. So I held my breath and took a big leap of faith - in myself. They did get louder, but I realised there was no way they could get any meaner. I had made it outside of the door to my room. There were now only a few doors left of which to conquer to reach the outside.

Although my words remained within never coming out, I began to place things upon my tongue; I had started to eat. Despite my many prayers, there was no escape from the cruel words which continued to eat at me. As I attempted to swallow, their screams would direct me to vomit. Remaining fiercely loyal to my enemies, I silenced any repulsion or gagging in order to keep their presence hidden. I wished so dearly to win my fight and take first place, but there were so many things with which to compete that I had not even made it to the list of winners.

Despite my failings, I continued to venture further out, into the ward, away from my solitude. I would sit in the TV room watching out the window next to me. The world outside was much easier to follow than the pictures and noise which possessed the ward in which I was locked. I tried to escape by looking at the smooth picture outside, and blocking my reception to the distorted images, and sound which pulverized my brain. But it was no use, after even a short time, a raging fire would surround me. I was so close that I could feel its intense heat which threatened to swallow me. Within crackling flames, I could not escape even the whispers, which together, created a roar around me. With the fear of being burned, I stepped through the flames my mind could see, and headed away from their touch, to my room. After cooling down, I would return to see how long, each time, I could withstand the fire.

***

ALMOST NORMAL

Do they really know how much I struggle? If I take a shower, do they know that each time I do this I must solve an intricate Calculus problem - when Calculus is difficult?

I fight to bring each thought forward while I struggle to understand the process before me. Sometimes I make a mistake and do things backwards. Despite the challenge, I struggle forth. Once the problem is solved, I can relax and sense a feeling of accomplishment. But only I know this. So while everyone thinks I'm healthy for taking a shower, I wonder what they would think if they knew that I had just solved a Calculus problem instead.

***

With each attempt my strength grew and my ability to withstand the volatile energy which had besieged me. It was time to speak. But the choice had been buried deep, paralysed within my throat. There had never been a choice; I had not chosen not to speak, I just couldn't. I choked as I struggled to awaken my dead voice. With a violent fight for their life, my words began to vibrate slowly warming my frozen vocal cords.

The ice soon melted, and I regained my

speech. But the ability to speak continued to feel awkward. Not only was I learning to form words for the first time - again, I was learning how to get out of the hospital. So as I practiced my words, I worked on the lock to open doors, releasing me from inside to out.

To get out, I stayed out - of my room. I spent countless hours sitting near the television where I could look out of a window of entertainment. Suddenly the volume of the TV increased and it began to disturb me. This disruption led me down a path of distraction. I sat thinking of its mighty volume, and how it was assaulting the room. Then I began to think of noise, and its significance to the balance of order. Suddenly a nurse appeared, complaining of the volume, and turned it down. I said, "Thank You!" Although most people could have reached forward and turned it down, my intentions had become so lost that I was stuck and couldn't move. Because of this I knew I was still inside, behind the locked doors.

Slowly with great effort, I climbed the list. Although I had not come in first place, I had won. They offered to unlock the doors for me, but now I wasn't sure if I wanted to leave; I didn't want to go to hell again. But given time to think about it, I was anxious to get home and I had hope that I was ready. Although I had unlocked the doors, and they had allowed me to leave, part of me was left behind. I was well enough to be let out, but I was still sick enough that I would remain inside.

Chapter Twenty-five

I returned to my apartment. I was safely in my home inside myself. This time, unlike every other time, I did not desire to venture out. Although I left my apartment to run errands, I stayed inside. I didn't choose to stay inside. My victory had left me so grounded that I could no longer get up; my mind could not begin to imagine going to school or holding a job. Now that didn't matter, nothing mattered. It wasn't that I no longer cared; it was just that I no longer could care. Meanwhile the additional meds were still gaining ground, and perhaps they could move at least my mind; maybe enough to retake my claim to the small lot of normalcy which I had possessed.

So I took the meds. Once again the weight began to pound my frame. As my end became larger, the end of my compliance became clearer. Despite this I continued to take the medicine hoping that soon I would be out gaining ground on my road to being functional. But I continued to wear the heavy weight of the medicine not only on my body, but on the supporting shoulders of my self esteem. The weight began to get so great that I began to hunch over the area in which I was still grounded; I was still inside. I continued to support this great struggle; the side-effects to the medicine which could not bring me back. Then one day the load was too much to carry. I stood, crippled like an old lady in the food store, engaged in a conversation with an employee and surrounded by noise. But that's all there was. Suddenly I grew more afraid than I had ever been in my life. While I marvelled with what ease I could converse, and track the conversation, I became aware of how frighteningly alone I was now inside. I ran away from the effects of the additional medicine into the arms of the medication which had held me unsuccessfully grounded before, and I embraced non-compliance. I deathly feared to exist in a world in which the voices no longer existed.

***

I have always been told that I should be normal. Even if this was not told to me by words, it was made clear through actions. With each forward movement I received praise, and for each flight which sent me crooked off the beaten path, I received a punishment with no end. So now I lie beaten from trying to be almost normal, almost something I'm not.

And since this is a fight which I must forfeit or risk death, I surrender. Although I did not win, I have not lost. So I leave with pride, and head to the locker room to be with myself.

Chapter Twenty-six

How was I to know that among the myriad of tortures, there would emerge a blessing? If I could not be normal, if I could not at least finish my degree, I was a piece of shit. Now I don't care. In fact sometimes I don't care about anything; I am unable to care. Although I may have given-up on trying to be normal, I didn't give up. But still, I find myself searching for feeling, but finding only that I am without. I thank God that the illness had led me to this place. Although at times it feels so foreign and uncomfortable and must move to prevent myself from thinking about this, I would rather be here than crucifying myself for not being normal.

***

I now sit comfortably against my tree, smiling up at the beauty which hovers above me which protects me from the burning rays of the sun. As *she* smiles down on me, I am reminded that I am not alone. I am only alone when I am outside myself.

So carefully I remove the thorns from my eyes, so that I am able to see the world that God had intended me to see. Although this process is not free of pain; I am rewarded with the beauty of knowing that I truly am special: knowing a world which is closer to God.

And as the wind blows and the tree sways from its kiss, sometimes I find that I have allowed myself to slip dangerously close to the sun's touch. So whenever I begin to burn, I pull myself in where I am safe, within the shade of myself; this is where I want to be.

So when the outsiders come walking by, stop, look and scream, "Get up!" I will smile softly, and remain quiet. It's not that I do not hear them; it's just that, this time, I do not understand what they are saying to me.

So I watch from the inside, as the outside passes by - as it must. I watch as children grow to independence, reaching up for more, perhaps a promotion or a family. And as I now willingly stand still for God, I realise deep within myself that I am now moving. Only when I was chasing the horizon, chasing a person I could never be, was I standing still.

And now that I am moving it's difficult to say where I will end up. Now that I can finally rest, the whole world lies before me ready to be discovered. The only limit being, of course, that I must exist within myself.

If people walk by carrying a welcomed

curiosity, I will still try to wave. Whether they see me or understand the gesture, I won't know until they sit down beside me and lovingly ask questions.

But if anyone does ask, I will tell them this...

"I cannot change who I am. For many years I was imprisoned in the worst hell for trying to be something I wasn't. I was finally released to feel just a little bit - of hope. And the only hope that I need now is that I can change people, and help them understand what I - and so many others - cannot change."

***

I cannot change the horizon. It will always be there. Before allowing another sun to set, I have released myself this one time from the unending chase, to finally rest with peace. And as the sun settles this time, I reflect, and then fly away to a better place.

ALMOST NORMAL

Chapter Twenty-seven

I did land in a better place - my thirties. Things changed in my 30's. I guess you could say I was reborn. My parents also called to see how I was doing. I don't know where or when my life began to change but it was for the better. I almost thought I was normal and my parents became my friends. I had never completely accepted being abnormal. I grew up wrapped in desire to be normal — a cocoon or metamorphous passed down by my father. The truth is that I would chase the horizon until I was dead.

To start with I got a job. Not just any job. I was now working in the group home in which I had stayed at during times of struggle. I worked the evening and night shift - often a 12 hour shift 7pm-7am. The consumer was now the staff.

For those who don't know, the group home is a transitional living space that mentally ill people often go to when they are not ready for independence. It is often also used as a safe place to go before hospitalisation. Consumers have chores and cook for each other. My longest stay was two weeks.

***

It's strange being on the other side - where do you draw the line? I can no longer associate with my own kind and the staff are hesitant to include me in friendships. Is it possible to be normal once you are labelled? So I continue in limbo and more alone than I was when I was just abnormal.

***

I worked with the consumers 3 years of my new life. I kept my secret identity to myself - I now was a super hero. I could read their minds and predict the future. This is only because I was one of them. And as a traitor I confessed to staff their behaviours. I wanted a way out and I would find that God would grant me my wish.

Meanwhile I had given up on love - single till death do us part. In fragments I existed. But love will prevail and there at my doorstop it stood.

His name was Frank and he had arrived at my door to fix my VCR. I didn't think much of him but I was a big flirt and lonely. We decided that we would go to the coffee house some time. And in time we did.

He was a younger man, my first! But our relationship grew from the moment he knocked on the door. It didn't bother me that he was six years younger than me. All it took was that one night.

It was a sultry summer night when he invited me to his dumpy apartment. He had moved out on his own. Not only he welcomed me but the scurry of roaches found in a furnished apartment caught my attention. But I became tired and lay down on his bed. All my intense paranoia subsided. I fell asleep and then I woke up in his arms. From the start I had trusted this man. Soon I would find out why.

My parents stood with open arms and let Frank move in with me. Soon Frank and I were a couple. Frank agreed that I should be sterilised. There was no desire to pass on the hidden demon to anyone. So Frank sat by my side as I awoke from the anaesthetic.

My parents started not only to call but reach out. Frank and I lived in their house in our own apartment. They could have denied me this wish but they were making an effort to save me from loneliness. How did I know that the illness would never release me from the solitude?

***

Even my friends don't release me from the solitude. They are too busy fighting their own wars. Each soldier marches through my life sucking the energy right out of me. I don't know if it is safe to have friends with your own kind and I don't think it is possible with the Normals. So here I remain locked up imprisoned in my own cell with keys dangling before me but just out of reach.

***

Not only did my parent's give us cheap rent they helped us move out. They loved us so much that they helped us buy a house - no longer it seemed at the time were we under their roof. We moved in and began to make Briar Cliff our home. I was grateful for all that my parents had done for us. I started calling them on a regular basis. But soon the autonomy would fade and I would find myself much more dependent on them.

It's an illusion. You think that owning your own property will set you free from the restraints of a generation gap but the truth is that you become more dependent. Things need to be fixed and as mentioned before we are not in the position to fix them. What you have acquired is one beautiful big burden. But the truth is there is no going back. This is your home and you will fight to maintain it. And fight we did. The way we kept the house and things we did were never free of criticism. Nothing would ever be solved - it was another war. But after hiring a maid, things improved. She was a constant in our inconsistent world. Not only did she save us from the fight she went to battle and twice a week she came to clean. This made my parents quite happy. We had arrived at a truce.

Now Frank and I grew as a couple. Frank was there when I was sterilised; It was a minor turning point for me. It didn't bother me that I could not give birth anymore it just freaked me out that I was now sterile - I was no longer normal once again. And the Abnormalities continued. The hives that I had once, continued. It got to be a regular occurrence. I would wake up covered in hives with my lips swollen. It was monotonous. I would say, "Hey honey I got to go to the ER." He would say "OK" and then turn over in bed and go back to sleep. But he was reliable; he was there when I needed him and supportive when I left for the tenth time.

At this time my parents helped me buy a car. The car from the past, although unforgettable was aging. I had failed; I could not keep the past alive. For some reason the mounting rust around the wheels cried out to me. It was entropy, the law of increasing disorder. There was nothing I could do. Not only could I not fix it but it could not be fixed. The past had run its course and only the future held what might be the past.

So I had the perfect house, the perfect boyfriend and the perfect job. I was on top of my world. Then God struck down with a mighty blow. After years on certain medications I developed insulin-dependent diabetes. No longer would my medical doctor allow me to work nights. There went my perfect job, my perfect house saved only by my parents, and the only thing left standing my boyfriend.

So they ask, who did you get your diabetes from? I say you mean what gave me diabetes? Absolutely no one in my family has diabetes. It came from the meds. And let me tell you that injecting insulin in my fat belly 2 times a day has already gotten old. Then I think to myself, do I have the fortitude?

Then somewhere on the way to normalcy my boyfriend cracked. He was one of us! That's why I trusted him so. But now not only were my parents supporting me they were supporting Frank. Without their support Frank and I would be homeless.

***

What should a parent do? Save a child from drowning or even from walking the plank? My parents allowed us to walk the plank but they were always there to save us. In fact I now realise they were there to save every step of my life.

ALMOST NORMAL

They may have neglected me but they never gave me up. I was a difficult child.

***

It occurred to me one night in jail - the hospital - that my parents never gave up on me. I started crying in the night as I thought about how much they must have cared but had never given up. Why did they ask I never mention the voices that I heard when I was five? I then thought it was the devil and that I was bad, and it was nothing to bring to my parent's attention. And I don't know what they thought when I couldn't go outside all that summer for fear of germs. But they stuck nearby. I thought of all this and I continued to cry.

They never disowned me. For up and downs there were always middles in which we could connect. From the earliest beginnings to the most current victory or defeat they were there. My love grew quickly for them as I realised their sacrifice for me. And just as I began to praise them for their love and support God would strike me down again.

Just when your love reaches an understanding it's time to become confused. My father needed open heart surgery. He had a tumour in his heart. I worried that he would not make it just a little. For my father was the superman I always knew. But when the second round comes around there's no way to shake the fear of his passing on the surgery table. And that's exactly how they told me, one morning at breakfast. My father had to have open heart surgery again. How would I make it without him? I would be crushed if he died. Once again like aluminium can, my fragile mind riddled with madness.

I woke up feeling hopeless today wondering what the next day would bring. My father was headed to round two - his second open heart surgery. How it is a man of vitality is smothered with fear? Humbled and fragile the man I once knew as a mighty warrior. You fight to place your life in God's hands. But we all are weak. The fear creeps in and you fight once again to surrender to a higher power. So I wait, pray and beg God to answer my prayers. Please God don't take him now.

However he survived round two with complications. He looked good and then suddenly I saw the bloated and puffiness of his frame and wondered if he would survive this challenge. But what will be, will be.

I have been wondering about my mother. She does not call the hospital to see how he is doing - only I call. I wonder if she's afraid to call?

ALMOST NORMAL

After another short visit we went for lunch. It was there that I found an uncanny strength emanating from my mother. At first I thought she was oblivious to my father's condition. But after visiting my father when death seemed to be his neighbour, depression hung like a weight on my Mother's face. She had emotion after all. She would be saddened if he passed on, but she had the strength to survive.

I felt so torn. The father I once looked up to was now below me struggling. And my mother that was for the most part, never there for me, took charge and became my role model. How I longed for my father to return. But this is where the truth set in. No matter how normal I could be, I could not prolong life and I would have to learn to depend on myself.

And now I find myself. My grandmother passed on over a year ago. She lived a good life and I pray from heaven she can see some of my earthly successes. Now my father is waiting to find out his future. Meanwhile my diabetic nurse is knocking at my door. Knock knock. I can't hear you. I truly believe that I will be struck down before I am old, so I evade her at every opportunity.

Now Frank's true colours began to show. He had OCD: obsessive compulsive disorder. Some of the symptoms I shared, but although similar, different. I didn't understand his rituals, but I did understand his torture. So it went on to the point that Frank, my love, could no longer love me. The rituals increased like a creeping vine through my parent's life. Now, not only Frank was trying to survive, so was I. And my parents were behind us both.

Eventually Frank just crashed. He no longer survived in the working world. He relied on me and my parents. It was a good year before he could call on his own disability check. Now we were almost free: both of us carried the weight of disability. No longer was it a family issue but a relationship with him.

His illness continued to manifest in him. His parents were poor and couldn't help him. He was on his own. But my parents continued to support him until the disability came through.

***

It is now I face my greatest dilemma. They say in sickness and health in many marriage vows, but I can't take it. I love this man desperately but I am weak and can no longer maintain the endurance. Please God make something move. If I don't have any help, I'm going to die.

***

Frank is on disability now happily seeking nothing. I drive with panic attacks in my car. I can actually see the demons in him when they take hold. What can I do? Demons be gone! Frank feels better once he calms down but that is because he has survived and I don't know how many more he can take.

I now know what my parents went through. How does it feel to have your heart ripped out as you watch your love ones tortured and captured by an illness? Seeing all that potential stymied by an invisible force. All I know is that my parents possess a greater human strength than I do. They stuck by me but this was something I could not do with Frank.

So now it is 4:30am and I find myself just depressed. How can I go on living a lie - a lie to myself? Frank is cruel and unkind and then he pours on the sugar. Would life be easier alone? I don't know. He stood by me through many things. Am I a lesser person for not being able to reciprocate?

I find myself pensive. Am I single or am I not? Just when I have made up my mind to separate from Frank the Angels appear and remind me of the loneliness in my world. If I am lonely now what would happen if he were gone. When he is sick I want to leave, but when he is OK we could never part. I'd rather die than make a decision. So I continue to be tortured by his demons and my own.

I could only hold the pressure so long and then it blew. It was a mighty explosion. The horizon trembled before me as Frank stood still. There was no way to reach him. Then suddenly the clouds rolled in covering him until he disappeared. Not even the search and rescue dogs could find him. He was out of my life. I could no longer toil with his illness. It had burned a hole through my heart. I asked Frank to get an apartment. Was that too much to ask? So I ran away and when I returned I remained steadfast that we were splitting. But love has a way and after one look at his smile my heart melted. How could I not love this man?

But I felt sad. An even bigger despondency took hold. How long could I withstand the demons until they took possession again?

ALMOST NORMAL

It's called community mental health services. The one doctor sees hundreds of patients. If you are not doing well, you come back in two months. You have five minutes to make your case. Meanwhile you are on the verge of suicide groping for a panacea. The doctor had failed Frank. But hope was on the horizon. Frank was working on getting a second opinion- at the university.

***

So I renewed my vows to a marriage that would never take place. The Government stole my God given right to pursue happiness so I would forever be living in sin. If I were to marry my benefits would be cut. So I resolved that as long as he tried to get better I would continue to love him. There would be no professing to be man and wife. This was considered marriage even though if I profess to be Jesus Christ it does not make me Jesus Christ.

Chapter Twenty-eight

And at last I found a beginning to my end. My death was claimed by a rebirth. The love I felt for my parents grew and the warmth I felt for them rose up within me. They accepted me. Even though I had a disability it didn't matter to them. They loved me and had always loved me. So the fight to be normal was no longer important. No matter how normal I could become, I would always remain almost normal. From now on I would chase the horizon but I would realise that there was no end. And the faith I had discarded in my trials would come back to me bringing the strength I needed to carry on.

So yes I had been reborn. I now carried an undying respect for my parents. I ended my relationship with Frank and moved away. It was a new start. I quit drinking and began to exercise. I was no longer oppressed by Frank. My relatives found a new vitality in me with every day I was without Frank.

I also worked a job for three years - a record! My father had also risen to his challenge. I also had learned to find peace in myself for every day and what it might bring but I cannot fail to mention that it was through my faith and rebirth that I found acceptance.

ALMOST NORMAL

On April 18, 2006 I asked Jesus Christ to come into my heart. I found that for all the blessings there were still negatives. But the blessings were now welcomed with joy and the negatives were accepted peacefully. And that's the truth behind surrendering your life to a higher power.

LaVergne, TN USA
24 August 2009
155779LV00001B/7/P